EXPLAINING PARKINSON'S

Doreen Jarrett

Emerald Publishing
www.emeraldpublishing.co.uk

Emerald Publishing

978-1-84716-423-0

Printed by Grosvenor Group London

Cover design by Bookworks Islington

Whilst every effort has been made to ensure that the information
contained within this book is correct at the time of going to press, the
author and publisher can take no responsibility for any errors and
omissions contained within.

Contents

Chapter 10. Welfare Benefits and Employment 89

Chapter 11. Living and Coping With Parkinson's 103

Introduction

A good deal has been written about Parkinson's over the years, and there are many avenues through which information about the condition can be obtained. Throughout this book, which has been revised and updated as a second edition to include findings new to Parkinson's and also rights in the workplace, I will be also referring to various organisations that play a major role in providing invaluable information about Parkinson's disease.

My own background is non-medical so it should be understood from the outset that what you read in this book is in no way based on medical opinion, it is just a product of research and personal experiences. My personal experiences have involved my partner's relatives and very close friends of mine and I have been deeply involved in all aspects of Parkinson's from initial diagnosis to living with Parkinson's and medication and ongoing needs and support.

In addition to this, I myself was diagnosed mistakenly with Parkinson's disease by my doctor (although I hasten to add this was an initial diagnosis and he referred me to a specialist who, after a few months of tests, and a deep brain scan, informed me that I did not in fact have Parkinson's). What this little episode did was take me through the initial phase of trauma and then acceptance that I might have Parkinson's disease. It was the culmination of all these experiences that prompted me, with the aid of my partner, to write this book.

What is Parkinson's?

Parkinson's is (one of) the most common disorders of the nervous system. Muscle movements are affected with the main symptoms being tremors, stiffening of the muscles and, overall, slower movement patterns. Parkinson's was first identified in 1817 by Doctor James Parkinson, working in London. Although the condition has been in existence for a very long time, it is now more prevalent because of the aging population, the fact that people are living longer. It is recognised most frequently in people of 60 or over, although it is also prevalent in some younger people.

Doctors are now far more aware of Parkinson's and the advances in drugs available to treat them have been very significant, particularly in the last decade. Research nowadays is focussed on slowing and preventing the progression of the condition and there will be corresponding advances in the types of medication available.

This brief book covers the diagnosis of Parkinson's, dealing with the condition in its early stages and explaining the condition to others, choosing the most effective medication for you, choosing diet and putting together an exercise regime, a discussion of surgical options and also the financial aspects of Parkinson's such as benefits and employment. There is a section about people who care for those with Parkinson's and many useful contacts.

Initially, a lot of medical terminology is used and I do my best to elaborate on the meanings of various terms. I sincerely hope that you will benefit from this brief but nonetheless important and informative book .

Doreen Jarrett 2014

Chapter 1

The Underlying Causes of Parkinson's

As was mentioned in the introduction, Parkinson's was identified almost 200 years ago. However, as with a lot of illnesses, the exact cause of the condition remains a mystery, notwithstanding lots of research, and a number of factors are seen as contributory.

The brain

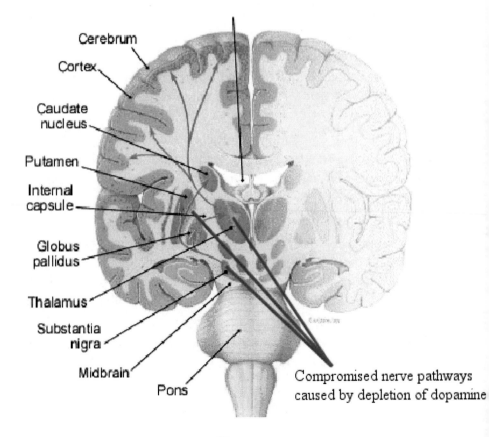

Cerebrum

Cortex

Caudate nucleus

Putamen

Internal capsule

Globus pallidus

Thalamus

Substantia nigra

Midbrain

Pons

Compromised nerve pathways caused by depletion of dopamine

The root of Parkinson's lies within the brain. Obviously, it is very difficult to treat the brain in a mechanistic way as it incorporates our mind and is our very existence. However, scientific research has determined that bodily movements are regulated by an area of the brain called the basal ganglia, whose cells require a proper balance of substances known as *dopamine* and *acetylcholine*, both involved in the transmission of nerve impulses. With Parkinson's, cells that produce dopamine begin to degenerate. When this happens, the insufficient dopamine disturbs the balance between dopamine and other transmitters, such as acetylcholine.

Therefore, dopamine can be seen as a chemical messenger responsible for transmitting signals between the substantia nigra and the next 'relay station' of the brain, which is the corpus striatum, to produce smooth, purposeful muscle activity. Loss of dopamine causes the nerve cells of the striatum to fire out of control, leaving the person unable to direct or control their movements in a normal manner.

The exact cause of this cell death or impairment is unknown. However, scientists have made advances in this area and one theory holds that free radicals, unstable and potentially damaging molecules generated by normal chemical reactions in the body, may contribute to nerve cell death that leads to Parkinson's.

Free Radicals and Anti-Oxidants

Free radicals are the highly unstable chemicals that attack, infiltrate and injure vital cell structures. Most stable chemical compounds in the body possess a pair of electrons. Sometimes, one member of the electron pair gets stripped away. The resulting compound (less one electron) is called a free radical.

The term 'free radical' means that it is now free to combine with another element to form a new stable compound. Free radicals can do a lot of damage by forming a chain reaction and breaking down other cell structures. A good comparison is that of the family unit. When two people join together and form a family unit, they are not usually available to other partners. However, if they separate the partners can go and look for another mate. Potentially, they can break up another stable marriage. This is the way free radicals work. When a free radical is born, it goes around the body looking for another compound to steal an electron from. While on the prowl, these free radicals can do tremendous damage to cells.

The most observed free radical chain reaction in living things is lipid peroxidation. The term lipid refers to any fat-soluble substance, animal or vegetable. Peroxidation means the formation of a peroxide molecule. These are the molecules with the greatest proportion of oxygen molecules.

Ninety-eight percent of the oxygen we breathe is used by tiny powerhouses within our cells called mitochondria, that convert sugar, fats and inorganic phosphate oxygen into adenosine triphosphate the universal form of energy that we need to live. This energy producing activity of the mitochondria involves a series of intricate complex and vital biochemical processes dependent on vast numbers of enzymes. These in turn are dependent upon dozens of nutrient factors and co-factors. In this metabolism process a very small amount of left over oxygen loses electrons, creating free radicals. These free radicals burn holes in our cellular membranes. Calcium penetrates our cells through these holes. This excess calcium results in cell death. This in turn weakens tissues and organs with the body, in turn weakening our overall immunity and resistance.

In addition to the oxygen that we breathe, the free radicals can also come from such things as environmental pollution, radiation, cigarette smoke, chemicals and herbicides.

Fundamental to having a healthy body is repairing the damage caused by the free radicals before it is too late and to protect the body's tissue cells from the free radicals before they cause mutations.

Antioxidants

Antioxidants are substances that have free radical chain reaction breaking properties. The antioxidants deactivate potentially dangerous free radicals before they can damage cells machinery. Most of these antioxidants come from plants and are called Phytochemicals. Among the most effective are vitamin A, C and E (known as the ACE trio against cancer). Out of these, vitamin C is the most effective.

Each cell produces its own antioxidants. However, the ability to produce them decreases with age. That is why (see the chapter on diet) a diet rich in antioxidant and phytochemical rich fruits and vegetables supplemented with additional vitamins and minerals is important.

Genetics

Researchers think, as do a lot of doctor's, that Parkinson's has a genetic link. The genetic material that makes us who and what we are is stored in our chromosomes. Chromosomes consist of deoxyribonucleic acid (DNA) which in turn consists of genes, which are the blueprints for our inherited traits such as the colour of our eyes, height and numerous other characteristics and conditions such as cancers and diabetes. A number of studies have taken place to try to determine the genetic link but most have been inconclusive.

When assessing whether a disease is inherited, researchers will examine family history. It appears that the genetic link is strongest with first-degree relatives, i.e. parents, siblings and children. The larger the number of relatives with a specific condition the greater the likelihood that a genetic factor has played a direct role in transmission.

When it comes to Parkinson's, however, it seems that the jury is out and that there are differing opinions as to the importance of the genetic link. Some families have a clear pattern of Parkinson's disease within the family tree. Multiple family members across the generations have the condition. A study of a family, the Contursi family, revealed that 60 family members had Parkinson's disease over five generations. Autopsies of several family members showed the classic loss of dopamine cells and the presence of Lewy bodies.

Parkinson's disease and inheritance factors

The chart below, compiled by Dr Jill Marjama-Lyons clearly demonstrates the risks of inheriting Parkinson's disease based on family history.

Person with Parkinson's disease in your family	Chance of getting Parkinson's disease
None	1-2 per cent, same as the general population
Brother or sister	5-6 per cent
One parent	10 per cent
Parent and sibling	20-40 per cent

As the table demonstrates, even if some family members have Parkinson's disease, there is no reason to assume that other family members will develop it as well. The risk may increase but there is nothing concrete by way of research to prove that this is absolutely the case.

Young-onset Parkinson's disease

Parkinson's disease is not solely a disease of the elderly. While the majority of cases are diagnosed in older people, it is estimated that about 15 per cent of people with Parkinson's disease develop symptoms before the age of 50. It has been established that the rate of young-onset Parkinson's disease is on the rise. Those who develop the disease prior to 55 years of age are considered to have young-onset Parkinson's disease. Very rarely, people under 21 will develop the disease, which is then classified as juvenile-onset Parkinson's disease.

Other factors

Research has been carried out on the influence of the environment as a factor in contributing to Parkinson's disease. There is no clear evidence to suggest that environment is major factor. Relatively weak influences have shown to be a possible factor, such as drinking water from a well, the proximity to wood mills, and the associated chemicals employed in these mills and also exposure to herbicides and pesticides, particularly among agricultural workers. However, such factors only contribute to a very small minority of cases.

Exposure to heavy metals, occupational exposure, such as copper, lead, iron, manganese and so on, increases the risk of developing Parkinson's by up to 10 times compared to the normal population. In addition, the iron and aluminium content is much higher than normal in the brains of people with Parkinson's disease.

Viral infections may also play a role in triggering Parkinson's disease. For example, during the outbreak of sleeping sickness during the First World War, about 15 million people were infected with the virus, and about 6 million of those developed Parkinson's symptoms. However, it was found later, during autopsies of some of the victims that the symptoms, although similar, weren't in fact Parkinson's.

Low levels of Estrogen

Some researchers believe that the female hormone estrogen may help protect against developing Parkinson's disease. This connection was supported by research published in the American journal *Movement Disorders* which compared the medical records of 72 women with Parkinson's disease and a group of women the same age who did not have the disease. The researchers found that the women who developed Parkinson's had three times the rate of hysterectomies, a higher rate of early menopause, and a lower rate of estrogen replacement therapy after menopause. The study suggested that estrogen may help to prevent or delay the onset of Parkinson's disease.

Caffeine and Nicotine

Caffeine has been blamed for many negative health effects. However, it has also been associated with a lower rate of Parkinson's disease. Numerous studies have shown that those who drink several cups of coffee a day have a lesser chance of developing Parkinson's disease than those who don't drink coffee. In addition, although cigarette smoking is very definitely harmful to health, ironically, people who smoke seem to have lower rates of Parkinson's disease than those who smoke. For reasons that are not clearly understood, nicotine appears to protect the dopamine producing cells in the brain.

This doesn't mean that you should take up smoking, far from it. Like a lot of studies, although the link between smoking and not developing Parkinson's was tenuously established, the fact is that smoking is a killer generally. So, if you don't smoke, don't start.

Diet and Nutrition

The exact relationship between diet and nutrition remains, like the other relationships, vague and controversial. Nothing that a person can eat, or not eat, has been definitely linked to Parkinson's. However, some researchers have shown that diet may help to prevent some cases of the disease. We will be discussing diet later on in the book, but briefly diets rich in antioxidants-such as vitamin C, Vitamin E and Beta-carotene-may help to reduce the levels of free radicals in the body, reducing the risk of developing Parkinson's disease.

Age related factors

In some individuals, the normal age-related wearing away of dopamine producing cells, plus the fact that we are living longer, accelerates the onset of Parkinson's disease. The older you get, whether male or female, the greater the chances of developing Parkinson's disease. The incidence of Parkinson's disease in the under 50's is less than 10 per 100,000 per year compared to more than 200 per 100,000 for those over 80. Parkinson's UK www.parkinsons.org.uk is in the process of funding many different research groups who are investigating all of the above areas in order to reach new conclusions in the causes and effects of Parkinson's.

In this chapter we have outlined the underlying causes of Parkinson's and also the potential contributory factors. As can be seen, there are a number of factors, however, research hasn't been conclusive and is still carrying on. Age and environmental influences seem to play a major role. In chapter two we will be looking at the diagnosis of Parkinson's disease and the importance of symptoms in recognising Parkinson's.

Chapter 2

The Diagnosis of Parkinson's Disease

As my own experience reflects, the diagnosis of Parkinson's disease has to be carried out very carefully and with certainty, as the consequences of a wrong diagnosis can be very stressful and traumatic for the person involved. In my case, once people, including in the first instance, my doctor, had convinced me that I had Parkinson's disease, I began to prepare myself for a life spent coping with the condition. It is therefore best not to listen to people around you, as everyone seems to be an amateur doctor, but make sure that you have specialist advice.

The main characteristics of Parkinson's disease

Although there are numerous symptoms of Parkinson's disease the main characteristics include slowness, general stiffness and an ongoing tremor.

Tremor

Tremor, which is the most common symptom associated with Parkinson's disease, is another term for shaking or trembling of the body. There are several types of tremor:

- Rest tremor, which occurs when the limb, usually wrist, fingers or arm, is relaxed and not in use. It ceases when the limb is in use.
- Postural tremor, which occurs when an arm or leg is held out against gravity, such as when holding a newspaper or book.

- Action tremor, as the name suggest this occurs when the limb is in use, such as when preparing food or eating.
- Pill rolling tremor, which occurs when rolling the thumb against the index finger.

Rigidity

Rigidity is a tightening or stiffening of the muscles. There are two basic types of rigidity, lead –pipe rigidity (the body won't move and is stiff, like a lead-pipe) and cogwheel rigidity (the body moves in a jerky motion, similar to the cogs in a wheel). In both types of rigidity the body does not move smoothly and there can also be pain.

The incidence of rigidity and overall stiffness will vary with individuals. Typically, rigidity occurs more on one side than the other and involves arms, legs, neck and back.

Bradykinesia

Bradykinesia is a general term referring to slowness of movement or speech. The term akinesia refers to absence of movement, which can also be a sign of Parkinson's disease. In most cases, akinesia shows up as an arm that does not swing when you walk or similar inability to move voluntarily.

Most people with Parkinson's disease experience some kind of bradykinesia, which can be experienced in a number of ways-from freeze attacks to difficulty dressing and walking to difficulty swallowing. These symptoms will come and go but when they are active the person may feel weakness.

Balance

Another very common symptom of Parkinson's disease is postural instability or problems with balance. Whilst this is not considered to be one of the major symptoms, many people with Parkinson's do have problems with their balance.

There are a number of other symptoms associated with Parkinson's such as light-headedness or fainting, problems with vision, problems with walking, weight loss, sleep problems and urinary problems. This list isn't exhaustive but your doctor, when assessing you for Parkinson's, or initially assessing your condition to determine whether or not it is Parkinson's will take them all into account.

The process of elimination

There is no specific diagnostic procedure or laboratory test to establish the diagnosis of Parkinson's disease. Therefore, a diagnosis is based on patterns. As the disease develops gradually, it is hard to be sure of a diagnosis until enough symptoms are present. Diagnosis is especially difficult in older people, because aging can cause some of the same problems as Parkinson's disease, such as loss of balance, slow movements, muscle stiffness and stooped posture.

Although there are no specific tests for Parkinson's disease, certain types of scans can provide evidence to support clinical diagnosis by measuring the ability of the brain to produce dopamine. These scans use processes called Positron Emission Tomography (PET) or Single Photon Emission Tomography (SPECT). These scans, however, are not used as a standard diagnostic test for Parkinson's disease. In my own case, I underwent a deep brain scan, which was an unpleasant experience, and it was this scan which provided conclusive evidence that my condition wasn't Parkinson's.

Carrying out the diagnosis

Given the difficult task of initially detecting Parkinson's disease, doctors usually have to carry out detective work, which is, essentially, a three-step process.

1. Assessing the symptoms

To diagnose Parkinson's disease, a doctor-preferably a neurologist or specialist-must carry out a review of the patients detailed medical history and perform a complete physical examination. The doctor will consider all the Parkinson's symptoms. In many cases, doctors will not consider Parkinson's as a possibility if there is not a tremor. However, as one in three people do not have tremors this is not really a very good starting point.

2. Consider all the possible diagnosis

After a detailed study of your symptoms, your doctor will need to look at the possibility of other diseases aside from Parkinson's. In the early stages, it can be very difficult to distinguish. Is arthritis present? Do you have a benign tremor? What exactly is happening? To make this determination, doctors should consider the fact that you may have another condition with symptoms similar to Parkinson's. There are a number of other possibilities:

Aging-this is the most obvious one. People tend to slow down as they get older. They walk more deliberately and experience problems with balance and also develop tremors, similar to Parkinson's.

Arthritis-this is another condition which has similarities to Parkinson's. Arthritis involves bone and joint pain, causing inflammation and loss of coordination. However, the symptoms of arthritis differ from Parkinson's in several ways:

- Arthritis is much easier to confirm with blood tests and x-rays.
- Arthritis causes joint pain and not muscle pain, as with Parkinson's

- Parkinson's symptoms don't respond to medication given for arthritis
- Arthritis doesn't cause tremors with muscle tone remaining normal.

Depression-depression can cause slow movement, stooped posture, weight loss and other common symptoms of Parkinson's. In addition, depression coexists alongside Parkinson's, making diagnosis more difficult. We will be discussing depression a little later in the book.

Essential tremor-many people, including medical people, confuse essential tremor with Parkinson tremor. Essential tremor is far more common than Parkinson's disease. People with essential tremor do not exhibit any other symptoms of Parkinson's disease, such as rigidity or problems with balance. Essential tremor is usually an action tremor that occurs on both sides, left and right while Parkinson's tremor usually appears at rest and only on one side.

Stroke-in some cases people with Parkinson's disease are diagnosed as having suffered a stroke because they present symptoms on one side of the body (this is most common when the person does not experience a tremor). In strokes, symptoms appear very quickly, whereas with Parkinson's they are gradual.

If, after exhaustive tests, Parkinson's is diagnosed, then a course of medication is prescribed to begin to try to establish a balance and rectify the perceived problems. Even at this stage, there is still a lot of uncertainty as Parkinson's disease is notoriously difficult to diagnose. It is only through time, and the onset of the condition, and trials with medication that the condition can be stabilized.

The next chapter deals with medication and the importance of getting the right medication, and also your role in identifying symptoms which in turn helps the doctor develop a successful program for you. Again, this chapter is not exhaustive as only a specialist can arrive at a correct dosage of the appropriate medication.

****

Chapter 3

Medication and Parkinson's

Having been through the initial, often traumatic, stages of the initial diagnosis, it is very necessary for you to build up a detailed knowledge of the type of medication that you will have to take for Parkinson's disease and also the side effects of that medication plus the effects of mixing medication.

In the first instance, if a doctor thinks that Parkinson's disease may be present, then, typically, a trial dose of dopamine-stimulating medication is administered. If, after this initial medication the patients condition improves then he or she is considered to have Parkinson's. If the patient does not improve then the doctor must consider another diagnosis.

Medications

Drugs that are currently in use to treat Parkinson's disease make movement easier and can prolong functions for many years. Overall, medications in use aim to replace, or to mimic, the missing chemical dopamine in the brain. The pharmacological treatment of Parkinson's is quite complex. While, overall, there are a large number of drugs that can be effective, their effectiveness will vary with the patient, the progression of the disease and the length of time that the medication has been used. Related side effects can preclude the use of certain medications, or require the introduction of a new drug to counteract them. Currently, there are five classes of drugs used to treat Parkinson's disease.

Drugs that replace dopamine

One particular drug that helps to replace dopamine is Levodopa (L-dopa) and is the single most effective treatment for the symptoms of Parkinson's disease. L-dopa is a derivative of dopamine, and is converted into dopamine by the brain. Doctors may choose to commence it when symptoms begin, or when they become serious enough to interfere with work or daily living.

L-dopa therapy usually remains effective for five years or longer. Following this, many patients develop motor fluctuations, including what is known as peak-dose dyskinesias (abnormal movements such as tics, twisting or restlessness) rapid loss of response after dosing and unpredictable drug response. Higher doses are usually tried, but may lead to an increase in dyskinesias. In addition, side effects of L-dopa may be nausea and vomiting, plus low blood pressure which can cause dizziness. These effects usually lessen after several weeks of therapy.

Enzyme inhibitors

Dopamine is broken down by several enzyme systems in the brain and elsewhere in the body and blocking these enzymes is a key strategy to prolonging the effect of a dose of dopamine. The two most commonly prescribed forms of L-dopa contain a drug to limit the amino acid and decarboxylase (an ADC inhibitor), one type of enzyme that breaks down dopamine. These combination drugs are Sinemet and Madopar. Controlled release formulations also aid in prolonging the effective interval of an L-dopa dose. The enzyme Moncamine oxidase B (MAO-B) inhibitor selegiline may be given as an add-on therapy for L-Dopa. Research indicates that selegiline may have a neuroprotective effect, sparing nigral cells from damage by free radicals. Because of this, and the fact that it has few side effects, it is also frequently prescribed early on in the disease before L-Dopa is begun.

Dopamine agonists

Dopamine works by stimulating receptors on the surface of corpus striatum cells. Drugs which also stimulate these receptors are called dopamine agonists. Dopamine agonists are used both as adjuncts to levodopa therapy, and also initially in early Parkinson's disease, especially in young adults. The side effects of dopamine agonists are similar to those of levdopa, although they are less likely to cause involuntary movements and more likely to cause hallucinations or sleepiness.

This class of drugs includes the older dopamine agonists bromocripline (Partodel) and pergolide (permax) and the newer drugs pramipexole (Mirapex) and ropinirole (Requip). You should avoid dopamine agonists if you already experience hallucinations or confusion.

Anticholinergic drugs

Anticholinergics help control tremors in the early stages of the disease. Even so, they are only mildly beneficial and sometimes the benefits are offset by side effects such as dry mouth, nausea, urine retention, especially in men with enlarged prostrate-and severe constipation. These drugs can also cause or exacerbate mental problems, including memory loss, confusion and hallucinations.

Amantadine

Amantadine (Symadine, Symmeterel) stimulates the release of dopamine and may be used for patients with early mild symptoms. It has some benefit against muscle rigidity and slowness and may help older patients who are unresponsive to other drugs. It is less powerful than levodopa and may lose its effectiveness after about six months. It may also reduce motor fluctuations brought on by levadopa.

Using medications safely

There are basic guidelines for safe use of medication, listed below.

- Always continue with your course of medication and don't stop taking it unless you have consulted with your doctor. Appendix one shows an example of a medication log which should always be maintained so that you can produce evidence to your doctor if the medication is, in your opinion, not having the desired effect.
- Always begin medication with the lowest possible dose and increase gradually.
- If you experience side effects from Levdopa treatment ask your doctor about lowering the dose of the drug and adding a dopamine agonist.
- When changing a medication allow two to four weeks for your body to adjust before deciding that it is having a beneficial effect. It can take several weeks for your system to adjust to the new medication or dosage.
- Stick to a regular medication schedule, most important as keeping a steady amount of medication in your system will help reduce the likelihood of motor fluctuations.
- Before you take any new medication, ask your doctor to review the existing medications that you are taking and make sure that there are no side effects from mixing drugs.

The approach to treatment, and the administering of medications, differs for younger and older people. As a general rule, people over the age of 70 tend to take levdopa. Older people have trouble tolerating dopamine agonists without suffering side-effects, including confusion and hallucinations. Younger people often use dopamine agonists to manage their symptoms early in the disease, in part because younger people experience fewer side effects from these drugs than older people. In addition, younger people often have more time ahead of them to manage Parkinson's symptoms, and many of the drugs will eventually lose their effectiveness.

Whatever the combination of medication used, stay in control, make sure that you medicate regularly and always request information about drugs that you are using, particularly combinations of drugs.

In the next chapter, we will look at current surgery for Parkinson's disease and also at the ongoing research.

****

Chapter 4

Surgery for Parkinson's and Ongoing research

Surgery for Parkinson's Disease
Over the years, surgery for Parkinson's has developed and improved, particularly so since the 1980's. While medication remains the first line of treatment, there are surgical options available which should also be considered. Deep Brain Stimulation is the more common form of surgery used on people with Parkinson's along with what is know as 'lesioning'.

Deep Brain Stimulation
In the late 1990's, deep brain stimulation revolutionized the surgical treatment of Parkinson's disease. The surgery involves inserting a thin wire and electrodes into the brain, linking the wire to a remote battery, and stimulating the brain at a high frequency. The electrodes are positioned in the brain; the wires run under the skin along the skull and down the neck, eventually crossing over to a pacemaker battery pack in the chest wall.

Deep Brain Stimulation does not reverse all the symptoms, but tends to improve symptoms to a level where they were several years before. The physical changes associated with DBS are determined by the positioning of the electrodes.

Lesioning-Pallidotomy and Thalamotomy
Lesioning involves using a heat sensitive probe to make a small hole in the brain that will alter motor function and relieve Parkinson's symptoms.

Pallidotomy

Pallidotomy is the most common lesioning surgery for Parkinson's disease and has been available for the last 50 years. This procedure can help relieve tremors, rigidity and bradykinesia (slowness of movement) by 15-20% and dyskinesia (abnormal movements other than tremor) by up to 80%. However, Pallidotomy doesn't help people with walking and balance. Pallidotomy is often recommended for people with Parkinson's symptoms that cannot be controlled with medication, as well as for those with disabling dyskinesia.

Thalamotomy

Thalamotomy can help reduce Parkinson's tremor and essential tremor by as much as 90% but does not significantly reduce rigidity or bradykinesia. For this reason, thalamotomy is typically used only on patients with tremor-predominant PD or severe essential tremor that does not respond to medication.

Cell implants

Research is under way to find a way to restore function to patients with Parkinson's disease by implanting cells into the damaged region of the brain. Cells from a patient's adrenal medulla (which normally produces neurotransmitter substances including dopamine) have been tried but little improvements in symptoms was found.

Mixed results have been obtained with cells taken from the brain of human foetuses. These cells develop into neurons of the type lost from the substantia nigra in Parkinson's disease. This is a very sensitive and intricate procedure and the results have been varied

Work is now taking place to develop human cells that can be grown in a laboratory and will produce dopamine, perhaps by altering the cells DNA. These cells may then be put into a special type of capsule that protects them but allows the dopamine to leave These capsules may be microscopic and suitable for inserting into the same area of the brain as foetal implants.

Stem cells from embryos

A further area of research is the use of stem cells from human embryos. These cells are at an immature, early stage of development and, with the correct genetic signal, can change into any type of cell, including nerve cells. This is what happens normally after fertilisation-the few cells that grow from the fertilised egg go on to develop into all the different types of cell that form a baby. Each cell in your body has the genetic information to become any type of cell, it just depends which genes are active. It is hoped that we can find out how to switch on the genes that convert stem cells into neurons for implantation to improve Parkinson's disease. This particular research is still at the early stage.

Growth factors

Growth factors are molecules that can be obtained from a variety of different cell types in the body. They occur naturally and are designed to encourage the growth and maturation of cells. Growth factors derived from the brain and glial cells (a type of cell in the brain) have both been used with success in animals and some Parkinson's disease patients. This research is still in the early stages but may become a useful treatment in the future.

Surgery is one option for people with Parkinson's disease. However, most people try to stabilise the condition with medication. This involves a relationship between you and your doctor. Establishing a strong relationship is of the utmost importance. This relationship must be characterized by trust and openness and also the sharing of information.

In appendix one I have inserted a medication log, which is the main way of compiling ongoing evidence which will inform the doctor and enable him or her to provide the best course of medication. The next chapter deals with your relationship with your doctor and also any specialists that you may see.

****

Chapter 5

Finding the Right GP/Consultant

It is a fact that many of us will place ourselves in the hands of our doctor's, or consultants, and implicitly trust them to look after us and give us the best advice possible. I am afraid that this is not always borne out by experience. The type of care and advice that you might receive very much depends on the attitudes of individual doctors, some of whom are better than others.

Whether you are in the process of confirming a diagnosis of Parkinson's or need to work with your doctor to manage your ongoing condition, it is absolutely essential that you choose a doctor that you feel comfortable with and that you trust. Normally, within a family doctor practice there are different doctors who tend to specialise. You must ensure that you find the doctor best suited to you. If you have any questions about your diagnosis be sure to seek a second opinion-don't just rely on the diagnosis and 'grin and bear' it. Don't feel afraid to change your doctor if you need to, it is your life and your well-being.

Right at the outset, you will want to identify a group of people who will support you through your condition. These will include:

- A general practitioner, i.e. your doctor, who will address your overall health care and needs and also provide referrals.

- From your doctor's recommendation, a neurologist, who will manage your Parkinson's disease

- A movement-disorders specialist if your neurologist doesn't have experience in this field. The neurologist will usually recommend such a person
- A physical therapist who will help you to develop an exercise regime suited to you
- A dietitian who will assist you with your diet.

It will be up to you to be proactive when establishing this group-you should take the initiative don't leave this to the professionals. My own experience has been that unless you ask you won't always get!

Of most importance, you will want people who have the most experience in treating people with Parkinson's disorders. This is essential. Never be afraid to ask questions about your condition, don't get sidetracked and make sure that you get the right answers. This is particularly the case with medication as, in the first throes of Parkinson's, medication can take some getting used to, with all sorts of side effects. It is this area that you will need to ensure that you get right.

These are a number of very important questions that you should ask a doctor:

1. Can you determine the reason I developed Parkinson's disease?
2. Do you have experience of working with Parkinson's patients?
3. How many patients do you see on a regular basis?
4. What are my treatment options?
5. What are the pros and cons of each treatment?
6. What short-term and long-term side effects can I anticipate from the treatment? Is there anything I can do to minimise them?

7. Can you recommend any support groups for my family and me?
8. Are there any non- medication options that might help? What lifestyle modifications can I make to help me feel better?
9. Are there any foods, supplements or over-the-counter medications I should avoid?
10. Where can I find more information about the illness?
11. Can you recommend any relaxation and stress-relief techniques?
12. Are there any clinical trials I can participate in?
13. What is your personal opinion about surgery for Parkinson's?
14. What is the success rate using surgery?
15. What is your opinion about alternative therapies?
16. Who will cover for you if you are away and I have problems?

Ultimately, as with any condition, it is vitally important that you communicate with your GP and take the lead. This will ensure that you get the best possible treatment.

One final tip is to always, if possible, try to maintain a record of your symptoms. See the appendix for a sample log. This will ensure that you can demonstrate clearly to the doctor what exactly the problems are and how frequently they occur.

Always keep a record of the medications that you are using and bring this to the doctors with you. Whilst it is true that the doctor will also have records it is important that you are in control as well as the doctor.

If you feel that it is necessary you should also bring a friend or carer to the doctors appointment with you as they can provide clarification and support. When you are with the doctor, you should not wait for the doctor to ask you about your most pressing concerns but you should outline these concerns right at the outset. Although doctor's are qualified they don't know everything and the dialogue between you and your doctor is a two-way process. Tell the doctor everything, even the most embarrassing symptoms that you would rather keep to yourself. It is very important to ensure that he or she has a clear picture of what is happening.

In the next chapter, we will look at the onset of depression and how it affects people with Parkinson's and how to combat it. I have also outlined a number of groups which play an important role in supporting people with Parkinson's.

****

Chapter 6

Combating Depression

Parkinson's and depression

When a person is diagnosed with Parkinson's, the trauma of that diagnosis can easily lead to depression. It is also common for depression to stay with a person, on and off, for many years. As depression can be debilitating, it is very important that you learn to recognise it and handle it to minimise the impact.

Factors contributing to depression

Living with Parkinson's means living with a situation where you are no longer functioning as you were. It is difficult to do the things that you once did and the knowledge that the condition is degenerative also has a negative impact. In addition, your brain chemistry has altered causing biochemical depression.

There are certain warning signs indicating clinical depression, as distinct to the common form of sadness felt by many Parkinson's sufferers.

- Changes in sleep patterns can be an early warning sign
- Changes in weight or eating habits
- Chronic fatigue or ongoing tiredness
- Apathy-although this is often a by-product of Parkinson's and can be distinct from depression
- Inability to concentrate or think clearly
- Withdrawal or isolation
- Anger and irritability

- Frequent crying
- Thoughts of suicide
- Apprehension about the future.

For most people with Parkinson's, depression is an organic illness involving both physical and biochemical changes in the body. It is very important to get the right medication at the early stages to minimise these changes. It is also crucial to ensure that you have access to counselling and professional care.

When it comes to treating depression, most mental health professionals rely on three specific forms of treatment, counselling or talking cures, medication (drug therapy) and, in the most extreme cases, ECT or Electro-Convulsive therapy. Usually, a combination of counselling and medication is used in the first instance and has the greatest success rate.

In most cases, depression usually responds relatively quickly to medication, such as drugs that inhibit the reuptake of seretonin (SSRI's) allowing the seretonin in the body to work longer. If you are in medication for depression you need to allow time for the drugs to work. Anti-depressants often take several weeks to lift the symptoms of depression. Medication should be used for several months during an initial period. You should work with your doctor to explore a range of treatments, until you find one suitable for you.

The importance of working towards acceptance of Parkinson's
When people are first diagnosed with Parkinson's, they almost always go through a process of grieving. It is essential that, during this period, you allow yourself to ride the emotional roller coaster associated with grieving. The five stages of grieving that have been identified are:

- Denial and isolation
- Anger
- Bargaining
- Depression
- Acceptance

Acceptance is the stage that you want to arrive at but you won't get there unless you have travelled through the other stages. The ongoing challenge with Parkinson's disease is that, once you have reached the stage of acceptance, you experience another setback or new symptoms that may require you to start the process over again. However, once you have reached the stage of acceptance then you will almost certainly be resilient enough to carry on.

It is very difficult indeed, in practice, to remain stoic when you are experiencing the ongoing conditions associated with Parkinson's. It is also very difficult for partners or those around you. The most important element here is having a knowledge of the condition and a future, forward looking philosophy that will take you through the dark times and allow you to focus on the future.

The importance of support groups

In the light of what we have just discussed, and the fact that most peoples personal circumstances differ, some have family, children and grandchildren, parents and so on, some people have no one, it is very important that people with Parkinson's have access to support groups. Within support groups you can share experiences and begin to understand that you are not alone with the condition. You can form new friendships and also gain invaluable advice about day-to-day living.

You will find many useful addresses at the rear of the book which can point you in the right direction, particularly in your own area.

One of the first ports of call is Parkinson's UK, formerly the Parkinson's Disease Society, address and website below and at the back of the book. This organisation provides a wealth of information and advice and guidance about Parkinson's disease. Below are some of the groups in alphabetical order and which are repeated in the back of the book.

European Parkinson's Disease Association (EPDA)

1 Northumberlad Avenue
Trafalgar Square
London WC2N 5BW
Tel: 0207 872 5510
www.epda.eu.com

Umbrella body for network of international Parkinson's disease groups, campaigning on behalf Of all suffers. Information leaflets on request. An S.A.E. requested.

Leonard Cheshire Disability

66 South Lambeth Road
London
SW8 1RL
Tel: 020 3242 0200
www.lcdisability.org
Email: info@lcdisability.org
Contact Customer Helpline on 0808 808 2236
email customerhelpline@lcdisability.org

Nation offices
Leonard Cheshire Disability Scotland

Murrayburgh House
17 Corstorphine Road

Edinburgh
EH12 6DD
Tel: 0131 346 9040
Fax: 0131 346 9050
email: scotlandoffice@LCDisability.org

Leonard Cheshire Disability Wales
Centre for Business
Office 3
12 Devon Place
Newport
Gwent
NP20 4NN
Tel: 01633 263807

Leonard Cheshire Disability Northern Ireland
5 Boucher Plaza
4-6 Boucher Road
Belfast
BT12 6HR
Tel: 028 9024 6247
Fax: 028 9024 6395
email: northernirelandoffice@LCDisability.org

Leonard Cheshire Disability offers care, support and a wide range of Information for disabled people aged between 18 and 65 years in the UK and worldwide to encourage independent living. Has respite and residential homes; offers holidays and rehabilitation.

Parkinson's UK
National Office
215 Vauxhall Bridge Road
London

Hepline: 0808 800 0303
Tel: 020 7931 8080
Fax: 020 7233 9908
www.parkinsons.org.uk
Email: hello@parkinsons.org.uk

Northern Ireland office
Parkinson's UK Northern Ireland
Wellington Park Business Centre
3 Wellington Park
Malone Road
Belfast BT9 6DJ
Phone: 028 9092 3370
Email: northernireland@parkinsons.org.uk

Scotland office
Parkinson's UK Scotland
Forsyth House
Lomond Court
Castle Business Park
Stirling FK9 4TU
Phone: 01786 433811
Email: scotland@parkinsons.org.uk

Wales office
Parkinson's UK Wales/Cymru
Maritime Offices
Woodland Terrace
Maesycoed
Pontypridd CF37 1DZ
Phone: 0844 225 3784
Email: wales@parkinsons.org.uk

Offers information and support via its local groups Has nurse specialists and welfare department, And funds research into Parkinson's disease.

Patients' Association
PO Box 935
Harrow
Middlesex
HA1 3YJ
Helpline: 0845 608 4455
Tel: 020 8423 9111
www.patients-association.com
Email: helpline@patients-association.com

Provides advice on patients' rights, leaflets and also a directory of self-help groups.

Disability Rights UK
12 City Forum
250 City Road
London
EC1V 8AF
Tel: 020 7250 3222
www.disabilityrightsuk

Campaigns to improve the rights and care of Disabled people. Sells special key to access locked disabled toilets.

Vitalise (previously Winged Fellowship Trust)
212 Business Design Centre
52 Upper street
London N1 OQH

General enquiries 0303 303 0145
www.vitalise.org.uk

Offers holidays at their own centres and overseas and respite care for people with severe disabilities by Providing voluntary carers. Also arranges holidays for people with alzheimer's disease/dementia and their carers.

YPN (Younger Parkinson's Network)
National helpline : 0808 800 0303
The young-onset self-help group of the Parkinson's Disease Society is designed really for those of Working age. There are around 1,300 members of YPN , many of them in their early 20s and 30s. Has a magazine, local meetings and conference every 2 years.

David Rayner Centre
120 Cambridge Road
Great Shelford
Cambridege
CB22 5JT
Helpline: 080 8800 0303
www.parkinsons.org.uk

Network of local groups bringing people with Parkinson's and their families together for support and help.

Parkinson's Home Care
Helping Hand Homecare
Arrow House
8-9 Church Street
Alcester
Warwickshire
B49 5AJ

Free phone: 0808 252 4191
www.helpinghandscare.co.uk

One of the most invaluable resources available to you is the internet. You can locate support groups local to you by surfing the web. In addition, Libraries are invaluable sources of information.

If you have, or you think that you have Parkinson's then there is a wealth of information out there to help you make contact with a variety of organisations that will be ready and able to assist you.

In the next chapter, we will move on to discussing the importance of diet and nutrition for those with Parkinson's. Many of the tips are universal and are common sense to all people. However, they are particularly important for those with Parkinson's.

****

Chapter 7

Diet and Parkinson's Disease

Whilst there is no special diet in use for people with Parkinson's disease, as with all people a well-balanced nutritious diet is an absolute must and will, in the long term, prove beneficial. It is a well known fact that with a proper diet, our bodies work more efficiently and we feel a lot more healthy. The upshot of this is that Parkinson's disease medications will work properly and more effectively with a well-balanced diet.

We (the authors) are not specialist dietitians and make no recommendations based on any specialism. The information contained below is based on good common sense and information gleaned from specialist publications.

Eating well with Parkinson's

Generally, Parkinson's patients should eat a well balanced diet, high in fruits and vegetables and relatively low in protein. The following represents sound guidelines for people with PD.

It is generally accepted that people with Parkinson's should eat more fibre. This helps to prevent constipation and helps to speed food through the digestive tract, minimising the amount of time that food remains in the intestines. Most people eat about 15 grams of fibre daily. Those with Parkinson's should strive to eat about double that amount. A useful source of fibre is dried fruit. You should also switch from refined to whole grains. You may also want to consider fibre supplements. Add these supplements to your diet slowly to avoid side effects which can include gas or diarrhoea.

In addition, it helps if Parkinson's sufferers drink lots of water. This helps with constipation and also helps with the respiratory system, acts as a lubricant and flushes waste through the bloodstream. It is a fact that some Parkinson's medication can contribute to dehydration. A good daily intake of water is around eight 8-ounce glasses per day. This should, ideally, be filtered or bottled water.

It is also well worth considering probiotics, or yoghurt. The 'good' bacteria found in yoghurt with live cultures and supplements help complete the digestive process, reduce inflammation and balance the endocrine system. You can obtain such foods from good health food stores and also pharmacies.

Like a lot of people with any sort of condition, it is best to avoid spicy foods. Some people with Parkinson's find that they experience violent dyskinesia after they eat spicy foods. It is best to give such foods a miss.

It is a fact that people with Parkinson's can be susceptible to thinning bones caused by osteoporosis. Foods high in calcium, magnesium and vitamin D should be consumed, timed to complement your medication. The maintenance of a healthy weight is very important and you will need to watch your calorie intake so that you can maintain your ideal weight. Some people with Parkinson's will lose weight (tremors and dyskinesia can burn an excessive amount of calories) others will gain weight as a result of the side effects of some medications).

Underweight
You may find that you are underweight and have difficulty putting weight on. Sometimes, weight loss can be due to practical problems to do with food preparation and keeping your food hot while you are eating.

The way you buy, store, prepare and cook food may need a little rethinking. It is recommended that you seek advice from an occupational therapist who can advise you on all aspects of food shopping and preparation, including kitchen and shopping aids. Here are a few tips:

- You should always try to plan your meals in advance, making a shopping list of all the necessary ingredients.
- When you are planning meals, you should decide how long you should stand at a cooker before you get tired.
- You should consider buying foods that are already prepared, such as frozen foods like vegetables and tinned fish, meat or beans. Ready meals will save time on all fronts.
- Keep well stocked with a wide supply of food.
- If you can, purchase a microwave, as they will save a lot of time.
- If you like a nap in the afternoon, keep hot water in a flask on a tray with a tea bag, milk, sugar etc. Drinking regularly helps you to keep warm
- You may be entitled to meals on wheels or home delivery of frozen meals. You should contact the home care organiser of your local social services department.

Dishes and cutlery
There are a variety of adapted utensils for eating and drinking which may be worth buying. However, it is strongly recommended that you seek the advice of an occupational therapist before buying expensive specialised equipment.

Specialised cutlery is available in various shapes and sizes and you should use large mugs for drinks, but only half-full. Two-handled cups can improve grip and reduce the chance of spillage. Special 'tumble-not' mugs are available with wide, non-slip bases and tall necks.

A 'stay-warm' plate might be useful if it takes you a long time to eat, or you could have smaller, more frequent meals. A damp cloth placed under a plate will stop it from slipping, or special mats can be used. High lipped plates are available that prevent spillage and make it easier to draw food onto the fork or spoon. Similarly, plate guards can be bought that clip onto your usual plates. Equipment is also available to help with opening jars and bottles. Information on all of the above specialist equipment can be obtained from Parkinson's UK.

Advice on eating and swallowing food

As important as diet, and the preparation of food, is how you eat. The following tips might be helpful:

- Take your time when you eat. Eat in a comfortable, quiet setting. However, if you feel that you are taking too long and your food is getting cold, consider eating smaller more frequent meals, or food that is easier to eat.
- Try eating in the recommended eating position. This is sitting upright in a chair with both feet on the floor and the arm that you are not using resting on the table.
- Try planning your meals for when your medication is working. You should avoid eating large meals when you are off your medication.
- Some people feel their throats tense up while eating and food sticks in their throat. You should try yawning before a meal to relax your throat.

Some people find certain foods more difficult to chew or swallow than others. If this is the case then you may want to consider a semi-solid diet. However, before you do so, you should speak to a registered dietitian or your GP who can advise you. This is because not all swallowing problems are to do with Parkinson's and it is necessary to confirm the cause of the problem before changing diet. You can also be advised on the best consistency and texture of food/liquid for you.

Semi-solid foods are generally easier to swallow than foods with mixed textures or very hard or dry foods.

Tips on easier swallowing:

- Try slightly thicker creamy soups rather than watery ones, or those with 'bits' in.
- Meat that is tough or chewy can be difficult. Try moistening this with either gravy or some kind of sauce, or try fish, which is usually softer.
- Try mashed potato, pasta or noodles as a change from bread.
- Try wholemeal instead of white bread as white bread can get stuck in the mouth.
- Try soft, moist biscuits, such as sponge fingers rather than drier crackers or toast.
- Having a drink with your meal makes chewing softer. Iced water in particular may help the 'strength' of your swallow.
- Good posture and a comfortable position when eating will also aid swallowing.
- Try taking smaller mouthfuls.
- If you wear dentures make sure that they fit properly.

Puree diets

If you find swallowing very difficult, you should again seek advice from suitably qualified people, such as a GP, dietitian or therapist. They might suggest that you try a puree diet.

Below are some tips on a puree diet.

- If foods are being liquidised or pureed, always use a milk based sauce or gravy, rather than water. This will increase the nutrients and energy of the meal.
- Do not use baby foods; although they may be the right texture, they are not nutritionally adequate for adults.
- Thickening agents can be added to liquidised or pureed foods to add back some of the texture. Suitable thickeners include milk powder, instant potato powder, custard powder or plain yoghurt.

Speech and language therapists, occupational therapists and registered dietitians can also advise further on diet, utensils and eating techniques. Again, there is plenty of information on the web site of Parkinson's UK related to diet.

A sample eating plan

As has been outlined above, and is also common sense, good nutrition in Parkinson's involves eating regularly, and also eating a wide range of different foods. Below is a sample eating plan with a variety of foods from which you can choose. Please bear in mind that this is only a sample and that you should pick and choose from what has been outlined.

See next page.

Breakfast	Fruit or fruit juice; cereal and milk; bread toast and butter (or margarine, soya spread etc) eggs, bacon, sausage etc; tea, coffee or milk.
Midday meal:	Meat, fish, eggs or cheese or alternative(consider cholesterol) Potato, rice, pasta or bread/toast;vegetables, yoghurt, custard or fruit drink.
Evening meal	Soup of fruit juice; meat, fish, eggs, beans or lentils, potato, rice, pasta, bread: salad or vegetables, yoghurt, ice cream and jelly
Between meals	Have a drink between meals, as well as with them, for example tea, coffee, soup, fruit juice, water etc. You can also snack lightly.
The main meals, midday and evening are interchangeable.	

Parkinson's medication and the interaction with food

Each of the medications in use with Parkinson's disease has a particular interaction with food. For example, levdopa generally works better when taken on an empty stomach. Therefore your doctor may possibly prescribe a combination of levdopa and carbidopa (known as sinemet) or carbidopa by itself (called Lodosyn). If nausea is a continual problem, then another drug may be prescribed to relieve these symptoms.

Controlling nausea

Given that nausea can be a problem with Parkinson's patients, it is useful to understand the best ways to control nausea. The following are useful tips:

- Drink clear or ice cold drinks. Drinks containing a small amount of sugars may calm the stomach better than other liquids.

- Avoid acidic drinks such as orange or grapefruit juices as they may worsen nausea.

- Drink liquids in between meals instead of during them.

- Avoid fried, greasy foods (always best avoided in all circumstances).

- Eat slowly, don't bolt food and eat smaller more frequent portions instead of large meals.

- Don't mix hot and cold foods. Eat foods that are cold at room temperature.

- Rest after you eat, don't rush around as this will bring on nausea.

Vitamins and minerals

Eating a well-balanced diet will provide adequate levels of vitamins and minerals for most people. Food contains fibre and other valuable nutrients, as well as vitamins and minerals. Essentially, if you feel that you are in need of more of a particular vitamin or mineral, it is usually advised that you eat more of the particular food containing them rather than buying expensive supplements.

In the next chapter, we will look at the benefits of exercise and Parkinson's disease. Exercise compliments diet and the two can combine to make you a healthy and able to cope better with life and your condition.

****

Chapter 8

The Benefits of Exercise and Parkinson's

Most people with Parkinson's understand the importance of exercise in the control and improvement of the disease.

Research has shown that there are several types of muscle weakness involved with Parkinson's, including weakening of the pulmonary muscles. Although those with Parkinson's will find it difficult at times to carry out exercises, it is important that a regular regime is adhered to.

The benefits of exercise

Exercise offers significant health benefits for everyone, whether or not they have Parkinson's disease. Exercise improves emotional and physical health, reduces risk of serious illness and increases overall energy levels. For those with Parkinson's regular exercise can help improve flexibility, reduce muscle stiffness and slow the advancement of Parkinson's symptoms.

Putting together an exercise plan

A well-rounded exercise plan includes three main components: aerobic fitness, muscle strength and flexibility.

Aerobic fitness

The word *Aerobic'* means 'using oxygen'. During aerobic exercise, your heart and lungs work harder than normal to provide muscles with the oxygen they demand, and you breath heavily and steadily to meet your body's increased need for oxygen. During an aerobic exercise, your heart and lungs cannot meet your body's increased need for oxygen for longer than a minute or two, and you are left gasping for breath, even if you are in fairly good condition. Simple aerobic exercises include jogging and running short distances.

Jogging and running may not be everyone's idea of fun and there are alternatives to this. Swimming is a very good exercise as are other forms of gym exercise. The important thing is to find an exercise that is suitable for your condition and temperament.

Numerous studies have found that aerobic exercise not only helps people with Parkinson's disease improve their aerobic capacity, but it also helps with movement problems, such as freezing.

When choosing an aerobic activity, you need to find an exercise that involves the rhythmic, repeated use of the major muscle groups, such as walking, yoga, or tai chi. When done regularly-for example three times a week for at least 20-30 minutes at a time-aerobic exercises improve the efficiency of the heart, lungs and muscles.

To derive the maximum benefit from these exercises, you need to work hard enough, but not too hard, particularly in the beginning and also if you need to lose some weight. You need to ease in slowly but surely. Your pulse rate (heart beats per minute) is your body's speedometer. It tells you how fast your heart is going and if you need to speed up or slow things down. Cardiovascular conditioning takes place when your heart beats at 70-85 per cent of its maximum safe rate. Your maximum heart rate is approximately 220 minus your age.

Dancing or exercising to music is seen as beneficial. Studies have found that people with Parkinson's disease who participated in music therapy-including rhythmic and free body movement-experienced significant reduction in bradykinesia (slowness of movement and rigidity). In addition to regular workouts, it is important that Parkinson's sufferers remain as active as possible at all times. This can involve any type of activity, such as shopping, walking around the garden or playing with children or grandchildren.

Improving muscle strength

Whilst Parkinson's sufferers are prone to muscle weakness and atrophy, they are not particularly side effects of Parkinson's or inevitable effects of aging. However, they do happen and there is only one way to combat this and that is through exercise. You can keep muscles strong and supple by performing strength- building exercises, such as weightlifting and isometric exercises.

Strength training also helps stabilize the joints and reduce risks of falling and injury. It has been proven that strength training also helps people with Parkinson's disease improve their walking velocity and stride length. Since most people with Parkinson's disease have some trouble with walking or gait at some time, it is clear that some type of strength training should be some part of your exercise programme.

Without strength training, you will lose muscle mass and strength. The average person will lose 10-20 percent of muscle strength between the ages of 20 to 50, and then another 25 to 30% between 50 to 70. However, this can be held at bay, or slowed, by strength training.

Flexibility

Flexibility is the opposite of rigidity, which is one of the defining characteristics of Parkinson's disease. Flexibility involves maintaining the range of motion in your joints, which can allow you to perform your everyday activities without discomfort.

Maintaining flexibility makes you less prone to muscle strains and sprains, and helps you support your joints.

Stretching is the key to preserving your flexibility. Begin with 10-minute stretching sessions in the morning and evening and work your way towards 20-minute sessions twice a day. You should move and stretch your entire body-neck, shoulders, waist, fingers, wrists, elbows, arms, toes, ankles, legs and hips-through their full range of motion in every direction. You should gently stretch and hold, then repeat two or three times. Only stretch to levels that you are comfortable with, don't overstretch as this can make things worse.

Stretch your facial muscles by opening your jaw, raise eyebrows, smile make facial expressions. Try to massage your face gently to reach the tiny muscles in your face. You need to talk to your GP or a therapist about a full list of stretching exercises, as you should for all other exercises.

Starting your exercises

For some people, it might be better to get a partner to help them begin exercising. This can be for the pleasure of exercising with someone else and also for practical reasons, such as someone to help you with balance and to assist you if you fall over. A very good option is to join a local group at a community centre or clinic. This might motivate you to maintain continuity. You can also share experiences.

Never do more than you can manage and never do any exercise that causes pain. You don't want to pull muscles or irritate joints. Organisations such as Parkinson's UK can give guidance on various forms of exercise and offer recommended programmes of exercise.

The next chapter looks at rights in the workplace and what to do if you are diagnosed with Parkinson's whilst at work or are looking for a job after a diagnosis of Parkinson's. for people with Parkinson's

****

Chapter 9

Employment and Parkinson's

Employment and Parkinson's

If you have Parkinson's, or you care for someone who does, you may have concerns about your working life. Work is not only a way of making a living, it can also be important for confidence, self-esteem and personal satisfaction.

If your treatment is carefully managed and you have plenty of support, it is possible to continue working for many years, depending on the type of job you have and how Parkinson's affects you. Speak to your GP, specialist or Parkinson's nurse about treatments to help you manage your symptoms and stay in work.

Sometimes, changes need to be made to make work easier, such as reducing your hours, changing career or taking early retirement.

If you are in paid work and care for someone with the condition, you may find that, as time goes on, combining your responsibilities can be challenging. You may also need to make changes to maintain your general health and well being.

The most important thing to do is stay as informed as you can about what your rights are in the work place and use all the support networks available to you.

Discrimination in the workplace

Because Parkinson's is a long-term condition you are likely to meet the statutory (legal) definition of disabled under the Equality Act 2010, or the Disability Discrimination Act 2006 in Northern Ireland.

This means that it is unlawful for an employer to discriminate against you because of your disability or because of something that happens as a consequence of your disability. Employers also have a duty to make changes to the way you work to help you continue doing your job. These are known as reasonable adjustments (see page 9).

These laws protect anyone who has a physical or mental impairment that has a long-term, substantial adverse effect on their normal day-to-day activities.

Looking for a job when you have Parkinson's

If you are looking for a job you may be wondering about how much you should tell a possible employer about your condition.

In Northern Ireland employers are still allowed to ask questions about health and disability before making a job offer and may ask you to complete a pre-employment health questionnaire. You should answer the questions on the form honestly.

But remember that the Equality Commission for Northern Ireland says that a response to a medical questionnaire, the results of a medical examination or the opinion of a Medical Advisor should only be one of a number of factors that an employer should consider in reaching their final decision about who to hire. In particular, your potential employer should also consider what reasonable adjustments, if any, may be required. They should then make their selection decision following an assessment of how you would perform in the job if these reasonable adjustments were made.

In Great Britain it is against the law for a potential employer to ask you about your health or any disability before offering you a job, except in very limited circumstances.

You should only be asked health-related questions when they're necessary for certain purposes, including the following.

- If a potential employer is trying to find out whether you need any changes or reasonable adjustments to be made to the recruitment process (for example, the time or place of the interview because of a disability or health condition).

- If you are applying as a disabled person under the government's 'Two Ticks' symbol (see the section on positive discrimination on page 7) or any similar schemes to improve employment rates for people with a disability. Note that the Two Ticks scheme is not applicable in Northern Ireland.

- For monitoring purposes. Potential employers can ask you to complete a form giving your race, gender, sexuality, religion, age and if you have a disability. Filling in these forms is usually optional and should not be part of your application.

- If a potential employer is trying to find out if you have a disability or health condition that would affect your ability to carry out an essential part of the job. For example, if you were applying for a job as a builder your employer could reasonably ask you if you have any condition that would affect your ability to climb scaffolding and work at heights.

- If they require an employee to have a particular disability or condition as part of the role they are recruiting for.

It is up to you whether you tell anyone about your condition. You only need to tell a potential employer about a disability if you think your Parkinson's may cause a health and safety risk either to you or to someone else. If you need your employer to make changes to the way you work, i.e. reasonable adjustments You may decide that you don't want to tell potential employers that you have Parkinson's. This may be because you don't feel comfortable telling people about your condition, you believe your symptoms won't interfere with your ability to do the job, you feel that, at this time, the fact that you have Parkinson's is irrelevant to your working life

On the other hand, you may decide you'd rather tell a potential employer about your condition. This may be because you prefer it when others know about your condition, your symptoms are quite noticeable and you want to explain these at your interview, you'd like to reassure your employer that you can do the job, perhaps with reasonable adjustments (if you think you need them)

If you do choose to mention your Parkinson's on your application or at interview, be prepared for the response. In Great Britain, an interviewer should accept what you have said and move on without asking you any further questions. This is because employers in Great Britain are not allowed to ask questions about health or disability before offering you a job.

In Northern Ireland potential employers are allowed to ask questions about your health, but they must be clear about what this information will be used for. For example, are they asking so they can consider what reasonable adjustments you may need?

Positive discrimination

Positive discrimination is when one person is chosen over another for a job because of their age, disability, marital status, race, sex or sexual orientation.

Generally, this is unlawful except in the case of disability. Both the Equality Act and the Disability Discrimination Act allow employers to actively seek people with a disability for a role in certain circumstances.

The most common forms of positive discrimination are the following.

- The 'Two Ticks' or Disability Symbol. The Disability Symbol is awarded by Jobcentre Plus to employers who make a commitment to employ, keep and develop disabled employees. This includes a guarantee to interview a disabled person who can do the job. If you are looking for work you may want to look out for employers who display this symbol in their adverts. This scheme is not run in Northern Ireland but there may be others. See the nidirect website www.nidirect.gov.uk for details of positive discrimination schemes in Northern Ireland.

- Adverts for jobs that say that the employer wants someone with a particular type of disability. This is usually because the role is working with people with that disability, for example the Royal National Institute for the Blind might want to employ someone who has a visual impairment.

If you are working when you are diagnosed or living with Parkinson's, you may be wondering what you should tell your employer about your condition.

Telling a manager about your diagnosis

This is up to you, though there may be some factors that influence your decision.

You don't have to tell your manager or anyone else at work about your Parkinson's unless:

- there is a health and safety risk (i.e. your condition means that either you or someone else may be at risk of harm)

- you need to change the way you work because of your symptoms. In this case you will need to ask your employer for a reasonable adjustment under the Equality Act or Disability Discrimination Act in Northern Ireland. Your employer will need to know how your disability makes it difficult for you to do your job.

Unless you work in a small organisation without a human resources function, your manager doesn't normally need to know that you have Parkinson's. You can just say that you have a health condition and you need to change the way you work (if this is the case).

Your manager will probably ask you to speak to someone in the human resources department and you may be referred to an occupational health specialist or other medical advisor. They will put a report together on how your condition affects your ability to do your job and what changes could be made to make sure you can keep working or remove any disadvantages you may have at work because of your disability.

If you work for a large organisation, they may have their own occupational health specialists. Smaller businesses may send you to a GP. The occupational health specialist or GP you're referred to will need to know your diagnosis and you should be asked to sign a consent form that lets them ask for reports from your own GP or specialist.

Remember that if you tell your manager about your condition, they must not tell anyone else without your consent, except in very limited circumstances. For example, they may have to tell human resources or other managers in order to comply with their legal obligations to you, such as their duty to look after your health and safety and to make reasonable adjustments under the Equality Act.

If they do tell anyone else about your condition outside of these circumstances, they may be breaking the law. This is because the Data Protection Act says that information about health is sensitive, personal data and may only usually be shared if you say so. If you do inform your manager and/or human resources department about your condition, you may find it helpful to ask for more information about their policies related to employees with a long-term condition.

Telling colleagues about your condition

It is entirely up to you whether you tell your colleagues about your condition. But the important thing to know is that you don't have to tell your colleagues if you don't want to.

Because you are under no obligation, you can take the time to decide what you think is best for you in terms of what, if anything, you tell your colleagues. You may want to think about things like how your condition may affect you and your colleagues in the workplace, how noticeable your symptoms are and what your relationship is like with the people you work with.

You may wish to discuss your decision with someone you trust outside of work or speak to others with similar experiences.

If you do decide to tell your colleagues about your condition, you may like to spend some time thinking about what you want to tell them and how you want to do this. You may want to tell them about Parkinson's in detail or you may prefer to be less specific and just let them know you have a health condition.

You may find it helpful to talk to your manager about how to tell your workmates. For example, you can tell them yourself or ask your manager to do it for you.

What are reasonable adjustments?

If you have Parkinson's, you may have difficulties in relation to where you work.

These difficulties may put you at a substantial disadvantage compared to other employees without a disability. By law, your employer must help to overcome or lessen that disadvantage by making changes to parts of the premises or working arrangements. These changes are called 'reasonable adjustments'.

These may include the following.

- Making changes to the premises where you work (for example, steps or doors).

- Altering your job, which may involve giving some of your non-core work that is difficult for you to someone else, like the occasional need for travel or work at a different site.

- Moving you to another post or place of work (see page 16 for more on redeployment)

- A change in working hours

- Giving you training

- Giving you modified equipment, such as computer adaptations, large button telephones or adjustable chairs

- Making instructions and manuals easier to use

- Using a reader or interpreter
- Increasing supervision

- Providing an automatic car if you need to drive at work

- Arranging with a taxi firm to supply taxis that will be paid for by Access to Work

- Working from home for some or all of the time, with the right equipment.

This list doesn't cover everything, because what is reasonable and effective will be different for everyone. Alongside yourself, an occupational health advisor or an Access to Work assessor is best placed to identify what adjustments may help you.

Making a request for reasonable adjustments

If you are having problems doing your job or parts of your job, the first thing to do is talk to your manager. An employer is only obligated to make reasonable adjustments if they know, or could reasonably be expected to know, that you have a disability. So you do need to tell them that you have a disability, but remember that you don't have to tell them you have Parkinson's if you don't want to.

Try to explain what part of your job is causing a problem and what that problem is. For example, you may have difficulties travelling to work on public transport during rush hour because you can't get a seat and find it difficult to stand for long periods of time. Or you may have problems using equipment such as a keyboard or computer because of movement difficulties.

You may also have some suggestions for changes that will help you. These could be starting and finishing later in the day, or speech to text software installed on your computer. These may have been adjustments that worked for you in a previous job.

Don't worry if you don't have any suggestions for what reasonable adjustments may help you. Your manager should arrange for you to have an assessment with an occupational health adviser to find out what your problems are and to make suggestions for how they can be solved.

If your manager does not do anything to make the reasonable adjustments you need, you will need to contact the human resources department.

You can also contact Access to Work and make an application for an assessment.

Take some time to think about what adjustments may help you, but remember that they have to be reasonable – i.e. something that your employer will be able to do.

If your employer is a member of the Business Disability Forum ask your manager to look at the website or call the advice line for practical advice on what to do, as well as information on what the law states. See the more information and support section for details of the Forum.

Workplace Adjustment Agreements

When you and your manager have agreed on some reasonable adjustments, it's a good idea to put them in writing. This is called a Tailored Adjustment Agreement or Workplace Adjustment Agreement.

The purpose of recording this agreement is to make sure that you and your employer have an accurate record of what has been agreed, reduce the need to rearrange your reasonable adjustments every time you change jobs, are relocated within the organisation or get a new manager and provide you and your line manager with a basis for discussion about your reasonable adjustments at any future meetings, such as your regular catch-ups or one to ones. (You should regularly review your adjustments with your manager to make sure they are still working and to agree and make any necessary changes)

You can download a template agreement from the Business Disability Forum address at the rear of this book.

Taking time off for medical appointments or treatments

You can ask to take time off work for your medical appointments or treatment as part of your reasonable adjustment agreement.

Talk to your manager about how much time you think you need. If the appointments are for fixed times and you know well in advance, your employer should be able to allow you to take the time off you need.

Sick leave

If you are too unwell to work you may need to take time off sick. Time off sick is unplanned. Under these circumstances you should follow your employer's usual procedure on reporting sickness.

This will include telling your employer immediately that you're not able to work. If you're off sick for more than seven days, you will need to arrange getting a doctor's 'fit note' to give to your employer. If you are off sick due to your Parkinson's symptoms and haven't told your employer about your condition yet, you may feel it's best to do so before they receive a fit note or letter from your doctor.

Returning to work

If you've taken some time off and your employer is aware of your disability, their policies may allow you to have a few days more for sick leave than other employees before they start attendance improvement procedures.

Some employers ask on their sickness certificate that you complete when you return to work if your absence was related to a disability. If you want your employer to know that you have a disability or if you think you need to change the way in which you work (i.e. reasonable adjustments), you should say yes to this question. This may mean that you have to see an occupational health adviser or other medical advisor who will ask you about your symptoms and the way they affect you at work.

If you've been on sick leave for more than a few days, your employer may ask you to see their occupational health adviser or other medical advisor before your sick pay entitlement has expired. If there is medical evidence that your Parkinson's means you are more likely to need more time off sick than other people, this is a good opportunity to agree on some reasonable adjustments to prevent you taking time of sick. For example, you may find it helps to work from home from time to time.

Access to Work programme

An Access to Work grant is money for practical support to people with a disability, such as a long-term health condition.

The Access to Work programme is administered by Jobcentre Plus or Jobs and Benefit Offices in Northern Ireland. It is there to provide help towards covering the costs of adjustments, which otherwise would not be reasonable (e.g. they would be too expensive for your employer). Your employer still has a duty to make reasonable adjustments under the Equality Act and the Disability discrimination Act.

Applications for Access to Work must be made by the person with the disability on the application form.

If you're in England, Scotland or Wales contact your regional Access to Work centre for more information or to apply. Contact details can be found at the back of the book. An adviser will then contact you and your line manager to arrange for an appraisal of your needs.

You can also visit www.gov.uk/access-to-work to find out more about the scheme.

If you're in Northern Ireland, you should contact an Employment Service Adviser in your local Jobs and Benefits office or JobCentre. You can find out where this is by calling the free phone number 0800 353 530.

You can also visit www.nidirect.gov.uk to find out more about the scheme.

Discrimination

This information applies whether you are a person with Parkinson's or if you care for someone with the condition.

If you feel you are being treated unfairly in the workplace, the first thing to do is talk to your line manager. Ask for a meeting and talk to them about what has been happening (for example, you may feel you are being discriminated against because the reasonable adjustments you requested haven't been made or you feel a colleague is treating you unfairly).

If your line manager is the problem, then you need to talk to their manager or the human resources manager. It's best to start with an informal discussion. Your employer may simply not realise what difficulties you may be having or be aware of their legal obligations. If you explain what you need they may be willing to make the necessary changes.

If you are uncomfortable about talking to your employer alone there are things you can do. If are a member of a union, you can ask a trade union representative to go with you or you can ask if you can bring a colleague of your choice with you to the meeting. You can also ask your employer to allow a family member or trusted friend to be there with you for moral support.

If, after the informal meeting, you are still unhappy, you should make a formal complaint or grievance. Your staff handbook should tell you the process for doing this, or you should ask for guidance from human resources department on the employer's policies.

You will also need to find out more about your legal rights. Your trade union, the Equality and Human Rights Commission (EHRC), the Citizens Advice Bureau or the Equality Commission for Northern Ireland should be able to provide you with advice. See the back of this book for more details.

Ending work

If you are dismissed because of your disability or because your employer doesn't want to make reasonable adjustments you may be able to make a claim for disability discrimination and/or unfair dismissal. You must find out what rights you have to bring a claim and what you should do next as soon as possible because strict time limits apply to making claims to the employment tribunal.

If you have been given a warning about your performance or conduct at work, you may be at risk of dismissal and should seek advice immediately. This can be from your Trade Union if you are a member, your local Citizens Advice Bureau or Law Centre or from the Disability Law Service.

Redundancy

The information on redundancy applies whether you are a person with Parkinson's or if you care for someone with the condition.

If all the correct procedures are followed, redundancy is a lawful and fair way of dismissing employees that the employer no longer has work for. Your employer can only lawfully make you redundant if:

- the business as a whole is closing

- a particular branch, office or workplace is closing

- fewer employees are needed to do particular work

- the job you are doing no longer exists

Remember that any periods of disability-related absence should be ignored for the purpose of selecting an employee for redundancy.

If you have worked for the same employer for two years or more you will be able to claim statutory redundancy pay. The amount will depend on your age, salary and length of service and your employer must give you a statement setting out how your redundancy pay has been calculated.

Currently you are entitled to:

- half a week's pay for each year of employment during which you were aged 21 or under

- one week's pay for each year of employment in which you were aged between 22 and 40

- one and a half week's pay for each year of employment in which you were aged 41 or over

The maximum number of years that can be taken into account is 20 and a week's pay is subject to an upper limit that is set annually.

When are dismissals not redundancies?

If you think that the real reason that you have been selected for redundancy is because of your condition or because you care for someone with Parkinson's then you may be able to make a claim for unfair dismissal and disability discrimination.

You need to seek legal advice as soon as possible, as strict time limits apply for making claims to the Employment Tribunal or the Industrial Tribunal in Northern Ireland. You can get help from your Trade Union if you are a member or from your local Citizens Advice Bureau, Law Centre or from the Disability Law

Service. Contact the Labour Relations Agency in Northern Ireland. See back of book for details.

If your job still needs to be done but you are not able to do the work for any reason, including because of your disability, this is not a redundancy. If you resign or are dismissed for any reason this is not because of redundancy, even if you don't have another job to go to.

An employee whose contract is terminated by the employer because they are no longer able to do their job or a suitable alternative job, even with reasonable adjustments, is also not redundant if the work they used to do still needs to be done by another employee.

Ask for redeployment as a reasonable adjustment

If there are no reasonable adjustments that would mean you could do your current job, your employers must look for suitable alternative jobs that you can be transferred to. Remember that the job might be suitable if other reasonable adjustments are made (for example, changing hours or location, providing equipment).

It is not enough for your employer to simply let you know about internal jobs and suggest that you apply. Disabled employees who need to be redeployed as a reasonable adjustment should not have to take part in competitive interviews for vacant jobs, if they are qualified to do them, or would be with a reasonable amount of training and support.

This is redeployment as a reasonable adjustment under the Equality Act and is different to redeployment of an employee, disabled or not, who is at risk of being made redundant.

If you can't do your job, even with reasonable adjustments, and there is no other suitable job in the organisation for you, your employer can terminate your contract. This may be a fair dismissal and as you are not redundant you will not be entitled to a redundancy payment. This is because your job still needs to be done and your employer will have to find someone else to do your job.

Retiring from work

Some people with Parkinson's may start thinking about giving up work completely before reaching state retirement age. This may be because they feel that working with Parkinson's is becoming too difficult and they want to concentrate on other aspects of their life.

If you do decide to retire, it may take time to adjust to life without work. Talking to someone may help. This may be a family member, trusted friend or others who have gone through retirement. A counsellor can also help.

Ill-health retirement and Permanent Health Insurance (PHI) schemes

If you have been paying into a pension scheme you may be able to take early ill health retirement. Whether or not this is possible will depend on the terms of your pension scheme. If you retire early but are still medically fit for work, the amount you get may be lower.

If you have ill health or disability insurance you may be able to make a claim on that policy. Remember, however, that to make a claim on such a permanent ill health or PHI scheme you need to be employed. If your contract of employment is terminated, you will not be able to claim on your insurance policy. If this happens you should seek legal advice as you may have a claim for breach of contract.

To make sure you are aware of all your options when getting your pension, it is advisable to talk to an independent financial adviser.

Work and caring for someone with Parkinson's

You may be working as well as caring for someone with Parkinson's. Paid work can provide financial independence and money to help with caring, a break from caring, social networks and friendships, self-esteem and a better pension, but combining your responsibilities has its own challenges.

Your employment needs should be taken into account in any assessment from your local authority.

Carers and discrimination in the workplace

If you care for someone with Parkinson's you are protected from being discriminated against or harassed at work because of your link to someone with a disability, such as a long-term condition.

This means that as a carer you should not be treated less favourably than another employee who isn't a carer, and should not be denied the flexibility you are legally entitled to. Any offensive language about your association with a person with Parkinson's should also not be tolerated.

Informing your employer that you are a carer

You do not have to tell your employer you are a carer but it may help if they are aware if you need to take time off to look after the person you care for. Checking your employee handbook or talking to the human resources department will also help you find out what support may be available to you at work. You might make this decision depending on whether your employer has a policy to support carers, or whether they'd be open to exploring ways to support you. Find out what's available before you approach your manager.

As a working carer, you are likely to need a range of support – such as access to a telephone to check on the person you care for. An understanding employer can make all the difference to whether or not you feel you can seek support.

Flexible working hours

You don't have the right to ask for reasonable adjustments but you may have a statutory (legal) right to ask your employer if you can work flexibly. This may mean changing your hours or working from home.

Your right to make this request will depend on your relationship to the person with Parkinson's and how long you have been working at your company. Your employer must give serious consideration to your request but they can refuse if there are good business reasons for doing so. Requests made under the statutory scheme will, if agreed, become permanent changes to your terms and conditions. To find out more about who has the statutory right to ask for flexible working visit www.gov.uk/flexible-working

Whether or not you meet the criteria for making a statutory request for work flexibility, remember that there is nothing stopping you from making an informal request to your employer. This may also be appropriate if you need a temporary change to your terms and conditions.

Getting support

If you are a member of a trade union, ask them for help. A local, or regional, union representative may be able to negotiate with your employer on your behalf and attend meetings with you.

If you are not in a union, you have the right to have a colleague attend certain types of meeting with you.

Time off in an emergency

The Employment Rights Act 1996 allows employees to take a 'reasonable' amount of time off work to deal with an emergency involving a dependent. A dependant could be one of the following.

- husband or wife

- partner

- child

- parent

- friend or family member who lives with you but doesn't pay rent

- someone who relies on you to care for them (for example, an elderly neighbour)

You should also find out how unpaid time off might affect your work rights, pension and working tax credit eligibility.

In the next chapter we look at the range of benefits available if you do decide to leave work or if you are out of work anyway.

****

Chapter 10

Welfare Benefits

The range of welfare benefits available

You will need to understand how the benefit system works and just what you may be entitled to if you are placed in a position where you are finding work difficult and you have to either work part time or give up work altogether. The summary below covers all benefits and makes reference to those that are particulalry pertinent to Parkinson sufferers.

Checking your benefit entitlement

The Department for Work and Pensions (DWP) and your local council are not obliged to inform you which benefits you are entitled to, which means it is your responsibility to ensure you are claiming all of the relevant benefits.

If you are having problems with benefits then a welfare rights adviser may be able to help. This is someone that specialises in benefits. They can check that you are receiving everything you are entitled to, assist with claims and help with appeals if anything goes wrong. You can find a local adviser by contacting a local advice agency such as a Citizens Advice Bureau. If you have a support package as a Parkinson sufferer then the person representing you will guide you towards an advisor.

Universal Credit (UC)

'Universal Credit' will replace the following benefits when it is rolled out in (initially, the aim was to roll out the new system in 2013 but there are currently delays):

Income-based Job Seekers Allowance
- Income-related Employment and Support Allowance
- Income Support
- Tax Credits
- Housing Benefit

The Department for Work and Pensions (DWP) was planning for all new claimants to claim UC in October 2013, with existing benefits claimants being moved over to the new benefit by 2017. However, watch the press for up to date details.

You can claim UC if your household income is low and you don't have much in savings. You can qualify whether you are in or out of work. This is important to note if you are forced to work part time because of your condition.

Employment and Support Allowance (ESA)

ESA is a benefit you can claim if you are too unwell to work. It was introduced in 2008 for new claimants, and everyone who is currently claiming Incapacity Benefit, Income Support (on the grounds of disability) or Severe Disablement Allowance will be assessed using the ESA criteria sometime between 2011 and 2014.

In order to make a decision about your ability to work the Department for Work and Pensions (DWP) will carry out a 'Work Capability Assessment' (WCA). This involves you (or your representative) completing a form called the ESA50 and providing the DWP with supporting medical evidence. You will usually have to attend an independent medical assessment carried out by a heath care professional from an organisation called Atos.

ESA can either be contribution based or income related, the main difference between the two is that contribution based ESA is not affected by your savings or income or the income of other people in your household whereas income related ESA is. You automatically qualify for help with prescription charges when claiming income related ESA. You will be given the contribution based benefit if you have paid or been credited with sufficient national insurance (NI) contributions.

If you do not meet the NI contributions conditions you will have to apply for income related ESA which is means tested. This means the amount of benefit you receive will be affected by most other forms of income and any capital or savings worth £6000 or more. If you have capital or savings worth more than £16000 you will not receive any income related ESA.

From October 2013 (however, check dates as this seems to be moving back all the time) if you do not meet the NI contributions conditions you will have to apply for Universal Credit on the grounds that you have limited capability for work, rather than income related ESA.

Job seekers allowance

JSA is a benefit for people who are unemployed and are available for full-time employment. If you are working less than 16 hours a week you can still claim JSA. Depending on your circumstances, you can sometimes keep up to £20 a week of earnings but you must be looking and available for full-time work.

JSA can either be contribution based or income related, the main difference between the two is that contribution based JSA is not affected by your savings or income or the income of other people in your household whereas income based JSA is. You automatically qualify for help with prescription charges when claiming income based JSA. You will be given the contribution based benefit if you have paid or been credited with sufficient national insurance (NI) contributions. If you do not meet the NI contributions conditions you will have to apply for income based JSA which is means tested. This means the amount of benefit you receive will be affected by most other forms of income and any capital or savings worth £6000 or more. If you have capital or savings worth more than £16000 you will not receive any income based JSA.

Depending on where you live, during October 2013 if you do not meet the NI contributions conditions you will have to apply for Universal Credit rather than income based JSA. (Again, check dates)

When you apply for JSA you will be required to sign a jobseekers agreement, which is a contract that will be drawn up on the first interview, stating that you are actively seeking full-time employment and setting out what you are going to do in order to find work. When a job seekers agreement is set up it is important to think about any limitations your illness or disability may cause as these should be factored into the contract.

You will usually be asked to attend a meeting to 'sign on' every two weeks where you will have to show that you are fulfilling the jobseekers agreement by looking for work. You can ask to speak to the Disability Employment Adviser (DEA) at your local Jobcentre Plus if you are claiming JSA and they could help you with your claim.

Income Support (IS)

You can claim income support if you are on a low income and not obliged to look for work because you are caring for someone or you are a lone parent of a child who is under five years old. There are other reasons that a person can claim Income Support but the rules are complex and cannot be covered in this summary. If you think you should be claiming Income support rather than ESA or JSA, it is recommended that you get assistance from a welfare rights adviser.

Incapacity Benefit (IB)

New claims for incapacity benefit stopped in October 2008 and were replaced by ESA. Some people are still receiving this benefit, but at the beginning of 2011 existing claimants of Incapacity Benefit started being reassessed using the ESA rules. The reassessment process is expected to take until March 2014. Your claim will not be reviewed if you reach pension age before 6th April 2014.

It is difficult to say exactly when an existing claimant of Incapacity Benefit will be reassessed for ESA, but the Jobcentre Plus helpline may be able to provide an approximate time frame if they are aware that not knowing is causing you anxiety.

Severe Disablement Allowance (SDA)

New claims for SDA stopped in April 2001, but if you were already claiming this benefit at that time, your claim may have been allowed to continue. SDA, like Incapacity Benefit is now being replaced by Employment & Support Allowance. The DWP aim to have all existing IB & SDA claimants reassessed for ESA by 2014.

It is difficult to say exactly when your SDA will be reviewed, but the Jobcentre Plus helpline may be able to provide an approximate time frame if they are aware that not knowing is causing you anxiety. You will be contacted by the DWP when your claim is going to be reviewed. Your SDA claim will not be reviewed if you are going to reach pension age before 6th April 2014.

Statutory Sick Pay (SSP)

SSP is not a really a welfare benefit. It is paid by employers to employees who are unable to work due to sickness. Employers are under a legal obligation to pay SSP for a maximum of 28 weeks if you meet the criteria. SSP is paid at £86.70 per week, but some employers will pay more. This is called contractual sick pay. You should check your contract of employment to see what you will be paid in the event of sickness. When your SSP is due to end, your employer will send you a form called an SSP1. If you are still too unwell to work at the point when SSP stops, you should claim ESA.

Working Tax Credit

If you are in paid work but have a low income you may be able to claim Working Tax Credits (WTC) to top up your wages. WTC is administered by Her Majesty's Revenue & Customs (HMRC) who have a tax credit calculator on their website:

http://www.hmrc.gov.uk/taxcredits/payments-entitlement/entitlement/question-how-much.htm

You may be entitled to an additional amount of WTC called the disability element, if you are disabled and your disability affects your chances of obtaining work. To qualify for the disability element you must:

- Usually work more than 16 hours per week
- Be able to show that your disability puts you at a disadvantage of finding work
- Receive, or recently received, a qualifying benefit – these include Disability Living Allowance, Personal Independence Payment, Incapacity Benefit and Employment and Support Allowance among others

Examples of a person who is at a disadvantage of finding work due to a mental illness may be:

- Someone who is receiving treatment or under supervision of a mental health professional
- A person who is often confused or forgetful
- Someone who has difficulty forming normal social relationships

If you are employed but suffer a reduction in earnings due to reduced hours, or an SSP/ESA claim, your entitlement to Working Tax Credits may change and you could be able to claim more money. It is important to inform HMRC of any changes in income or number of working hours so they can adjust your payment accordingly.

Disability Living Allowance (DLA) and Personal Independence Payment (PIP)

Disability Living Allowance (DLA) is a benefit for people with disabilities who need help with their personal care and/or help getting around. It has two components: a care component, which could be paid at one of three rates (lower, middle and higher); and a mobility component which has two rates (lower and higher). If you have both care and mobility needs you may receive payment for both components

DLA can be paid on top of Income Support, Employment and Support Allowance, Jobseekers Allowance and other benefits and will not reduce the amount you get. In some cases getting an award of DLA can actually increase the amount you get in other benefits. You can claim DLA regardless of your employment status.

From 8th April 2013, a new benefit called the Personal Independence Payment (PIP) was introduced to replace DLA. Initially, only new claimants in selected parts of the North of

England will need to claim PIP. However, the DWP is hoping that from July, all new claimants will claim PIP. Most existing DLA claimants with an indefinite award will not be affected until 2015 unless their circumstances changed after Oct 2013.

Housing Benefit

If you are on a low income and live in rented accommodation you may be able to claim Housing Benefit (HB) to help with the cost of rent. You can claim HB if you live in a property owned by a close relative as long as they do not live in the same household; however the rules can be complicated so it is recommended that you speak to a welfare rights adviser before claiming housing benefit for a property owned by a family member.

Council or housing association property

If your only income is from means tested benefits and you live in a property owned by the local authority or housing association your HB will usually cover the whole of your rent. If however you have additional income you may only get part of the rent paid, in which case you will be responsible for paying the shortfall. You may also have to top up your housing benefit if:

- Part of your rent pays for bills or services that are not covered by HB (such as electricity, meals or laundry services)
- You have a non-dependant living with you (a non-dependant may be an adult child, friend or relative who will be expected to contribute towards the rent)

You may also have your housing benefit reduced if you have more bedrooms in your property than the government thinks that you need. This has, unofficially, been called the 'bedroom tax'

If you are under-occupying one bedroom then your housing benefit will be reduced by 14%. If you are under-occupying more than one bedroom, your housing benefit will be reduced by 25%.

You will not be regarded as under-occupying one of your bedrooms if you need that extra bedroom for a carer to stay overnight to provide care for you. A carer would actually have to do this regularly in order for you to claim the exemption. It is not necessary for you to claim DLA or PIP in order to show that you need a carer to provide this care as long as you have other evidence.
If you are affected by the 'bedroom tax', you have the following options:

- Move House
- Take in a lodger
- Apply for 'discretionary housing payments' from your local council
- Increase your hours of work
- Get a benefits check to make sure you are receiving everything you are entitled to
- Pay the difference out of your benefits or other income if you can afford to do this

Local Housing Allowance (LHA)
If you live in a property or room that is rented from a private landlord Local Housing Allowance rules are used to work out how much housing benefit you get. The LHA rates depend on where you live, the number of people in your household and the size of your accommodation. This can range from a single room in a shared house to a property with four bedrooms.

Changes to housing benefit regulations in April 2011 means the local housing allowance size criteria can be increased for a person who has an established need for overnight care, is actually receiving that care, and has an additional room in their property. This means that you may be able to claim housing benefit for a property with an additional room if you have a non-resident carer that regularly needs to stay overnight.

From January 1st 2012 people under 35 have had their benefit restricted to the shared room rate. However some people will not be affected by the changes. The rules will not apply to you if:

- You get the middle or higher rate care component of Disability Living Allowance and no-one receives Carer's Allowance for you.
- You live with someone else (for example, a partner, child, elderly relative, friend or grown-up child); who is part of your household.
- You rent from a Local Authority or housing association.
- You live in supported housing provided by a housing association, registered charity or voluntary organisation and get a package of care or support from your landlord (or from somebody else on behalf of your landlord).
- Your private tenancy began before January 1989.
- You need an extra bedroom for a carer who does not live with you but who provides you with overnight care.
- You are under 22 and have been in the care of a local authority since the age of 16, or have been accommodated by a local authority since the age of 16.
- You have lived in a hostel for homeless people or a hostel that provides rehabilitation and resettlement within the community for at least three months. You must have received resettlement support to help you live in the community.

Support for Mortgage Interest (SMI)

If you live in a mortgaged property and you are claiming either income based ESA, Income Support or income based Jobseekers Allowance, you may be entitled to help with your mortgage payments through a benefit called Support for Mortgage Interest (SMI).

There is a 13 week waiting period from the time you claim until you get your first payment and payments will usually be made directly to your mortgage lender. SMI will only help with the interest portion of a mortgage up to the value of £200,000; it will not help pay back the amount you borrowed. The rate that SMI is paid at is based on the Bank of England's standard interest rate. You can find out how much the rate is at any time by checking 'support for mortgage interest' webpage at www.gov.uk.

If you do not have an interest-only mortgage you will either have to make up the shortfall on the actual mortgage payments to ensure you do not go into arrears, or come to a satisfactory arrangement with your lender such as switching to an interest-only mortgage. To apply for this benefit or to ask further questions you should contact Jobcentre Plus or the Pension Service. Their contact details are at the end of this section. When Universal Credit is introduced, it will include additional payments to meet mortgage interest costs.

Council Tax Support and Discounts

If you are liable for council tax and on a low income then you may be entitled to help with your council tax through Council Tax Support. This scheme replaced the national Council Tax Benefit on 1st April 2013. Council Tax Support is administered by your local authority through their local scheme, and may cover either part or your entire council tax bill depending on your household income. How much help you can get with your council tax will depend on your local scheme. However, the government has reduced the money available to local authorities by 10% and so it is likely that many working age people will have to contribute towards their council tax in order to make up the difference. It is important to ensure that your council tax bill is correct. If you are living alone or you are very unwell, you may be able to get your bill reduced.

Single person's discount

If you are the only adult living in a property you should be receiving a 'single person's discount' on your council tax bill, this will reduce the bill by 25%. You will also receive this discount if you are not the only adult, but the other people you live with are not liable to pay council tax because, for example they are students or exempt due to a 'severe mental impairment'.

Exemption due to severe mental impairment

The council tax rules say that a person is exempt from council tax if they have a 'severe mental impairment'. It states that 'a person is severely mentally impaired if he has a severe impairment of intelligence and social functioning (however caused) which appears to be permanent'.

To qualify for the exemption you must obtain confirmation from a doctor stating that you are severely mentally impaired and receive one of the following benefits:

- DLA with the middle or highest rate care component
- Personal Independence Payment Daily Living Component (standard or enhanced rate)
- Attendance Allowance
- Severe Disablement Allowance
- Employment and Support Allowance
- Incapacity Benefit

- Income Support or Jobseekers Allowance with a disability premium
- Working Tax Credit with the disability element

Disabled band reduction scheme

If you or a person that lives with you has a disability that means they require additional space, it may be possible to get the council tax bill reduced to the price of the next band down. So if, for example your property is in band C, you would be charged the band B rate.

To qualify for the disabled band reduction you would have to show that the property is the main residence of at least one disabled person. The property must also have an additional room to meet the needs of the disabled person (if the room is not a kitchen or bathroom it must be for the predominant use of the disabled person); or additional space to allow for wheelchair use.

If you think you should qualify for a band reduction, you should contact the local authority that issues your council tax bill.

The Social Fund

From April 2013, the discretionary social fund was disbanded. 'Crisis loans' and 'community care grants' will no longer be available. 'Budgeting loans' will continue to be available until they are replaced by 'budgeting advances' under the new Universal Credit scheme.

Crisis loans used to be very helpful to people who were experiencing a delay in the payment of their benefits for some reason. To replace crisis loans, the DWP can now provide 'short-term advances' to provide you with some money if you're having to wait for your benefits to be paid. The short-term advance will have to be paid back, just like a crisis loan.

Local authorities have been given the discretion to set up schemes to replace 'community care grants' if they would like to. Some local authorities may not set up schemes at all, and the ones that do may choose to do things very differently. We hope to be able to provide more information about this when we find out more about what local authorities are doing.

****

Chapter 11

Living and Coping with Parkinson's Disease- General Advice

When a person first receives a diagnosis of Parkinson's disease, it can be very stressful and also confusing, both for the individual and family and friends. It is crucial, at the outset, that advice and information is available.

One of the most important factors in the life of someone with Parkinson's disease, particularly someone who has been newly diagnosed, is that of ongoing support. There is a lot of support out there, not least the umbrella groups such as Parkinson's UK who can be contacted on 0808 800 0303 e mail hello@parkinsons.org.uk or online at www. parkinsons.org.uk.

In addition, there are Parkinson's disease nurse specialists who are community based or based in a hospital. Their numbers have expanded over the years although there is not yet one in every area. They are registered nurses who have specialised in the area of Parkinson's disease and they have broad experience in neurology or the care of elderly people. Their work involves assessing individual care needs, enhancing and promoting quality of life and preventing, or at least minimising the complications associated with Parkinson's disease. Typical complications can include problems with mobility, urinary problems, depression, and the side effects of medication.

Therapies for Parkinson's disease

Parkinson's disease can interfere, to a greater or lesser extent, with many day-to-day activities. The aim of therapies is to ease these difficulties by helping you to learn the knowledge and skills that you will need to continue with a normal life. There are three main therapies available, physiotherapy, occupational therapy and speech and language therapy.

Physiotherapy

A physiotherapist will assess your needs by looking at the difficulties that you have with movement and general mobility. The aim of the physiotherapist is to help you achieve the greatest level of activity possible. They will teach you how to manage the physical problems associated with Parkinson's disease.

Beware of those who call themselves physiotherapists. A Qualified physiotherapist will be a member of the Chartered Society of Physiotherapists. Each person will specialise in a different area of physiotherapy, as with most other professions and not all physiotherapists have the required expertise in neurological disorders. Physiotherapists interested in neurological disorders will be senior practitioners and will often be termed neurophysiotherapists.

Physiotherapy will help you move more normally and with less effort. Physiotherapy is not about routine exercise, as has already been outlined in this book, but about learning skills and techniques to assist you with coping with problems that arise with the onset and development of the disease. Certain basic tasks, which you have found easy all your life, such as tying a tie or doing up your shoelaces can become a chore when you have Parkinson's. Physiotherapy will teach you certain techniques and provide learning strategies, such as talking through a task while doing it or relying on visual targets to improve performance. These approaches are known as cueing.

Stiffness and poor posture also comes with Parkinson's. Muscles and joints will stiffen up over time making it increasingly harder to walk and relax. Physiotherapists can help to relieve this muscle and joint stiffness. Physiotherapists can also advise you about appropriate exercises that will help you, such as swimming or the Alexander technique.

Occupational therapy

Occupational therapists will assist you in those daily aspects of life that have become increasingly more difficult, such as looking after yourself and others, and also with work and leisure. It can also be difficult for you to travel where you want, because of mobility problems. Occupational therapists will work with you to improve your life by identifying areas of particular difficulty and devising a programme specifically for you to help you overcome these problems. A qualified occupational therapist will be state registered and have a degree (BSc (Hons) OT) or diploma (DipCot). As with physiotherapists occupational therapists specialise in different areas. These occupational therapists who have specialised in neurological disorders might be members of NANOT (National Association of Neurological OT's) or have done some further specialised training after initially qualifying as an occupational therapist.

Speech and language therapists

A speech and language therapist will work with Parkinson's sufferers and also, where necessary, with family or carers. They will identify where the difficulties impact on lifestyle, such as using the telephone or when conversing in shops or at work. Therapy will include exercises that work on improving voice loudness and intelligibility of speech generally. Communication can be affected by the types of swallowing difficulties encountered by people with Parkinson's, which include difficulties controlling saliva, difficulty chewing harder foods and problems with swallowing generally. Some may experience coughing or choking episodes while eating. A speech and language therapist will assess swallowing problems and provide advice on the easiest food and drinks and also the safest approach to eating and drinking. It is highly advisable to see a therapist as soon as possible after your initial diagnosis of Parkinson's. Your family doctor or consultant will usually make the referral to see a therapist

Driving and Parkinson's

A diagnosis of Parkinson's does not always mean that you will have to cease driving. However, you must by law inform the Driver and Vehicle Licensing Agency (DVLA). You can continue to drive after informing the DVLA until they inform you other wise. If you or your family or friends have any concerns, however, you should stop driving and discuss the matter with your doctor.

The DVLA assesses each case individually and may issue either a restricted licence, (restricted to a number of years or to a vehicle with adaptations) or an unrestricted licence. Both of these will allow you to continue driving once you have been diagnosed with Parkinson's. However, the DVLA can also decide that you should not be allowed to drive for a specified period. If you are not happy with the DVLA's decision then you can appeal asking them to reconsider or you can appeal in a magistrate's court.

When you contact the DVLA, you will need to complete two forms, PK1 'Medical in confidence' available from the DirectGov website and a shorter medical questionnaire detailing your symptoms and you may be required to undergo further medical assessment and possibly retake the practical part of the driving test. Medicals and driving tests are free to those newly diagnosed with Parkinson's. A more detailed booklet is available from www.parkinsons.org.uk.

Parkinson's medication and driving

The side effects that some people might experience from their medication can affect driving. Dopamine agonists can cause drowsiness, sometime severe. You need to be aware of this and consult the literature about side effects provided with your medication. You can also get advice from your doctor.

Mobility centres and driving assessment.

Mobility centres provide information and advice on driving for any person who is disabled and uses a car, either as a driver or a passenger. They will also offer assessments on your ability to drive a vehicle. There are a number of mobility centres in the UK, again information can be obtained from the DVLA website or from www. parkinsons.org.uk.

Priority parking and the Blue Badge Scheme

You may qualify for parking concessions through the Blue Badge Scheme if you have a severe disability and also qualify for the higher rate of the mobility component of the Disability Living Allowance (see chapter on benefits). The Blue Badge Scheme enables people who have certain disabilities to park closer to shops and the services that they need to get to. The badge applies whether they are driver or passenger in a vehicle. More information can be obtained from the DirectGov website www.directgov.co.uk. In addition to the above, if you are disabled and qualify for DLA or the War Pensioners Mobility Supplement you may also be eligible for a car tax exemption.

Car insurance and Parkinson's

If you have been diagnosed with Parkinson's you should inform your car insurance company as any changes in your health may affect your ability to drive and render your policy invalid. It is also an offence under the Road Traffic Act not to inform your insurer of changes of circumstances. You must also inform your insurers about any adaptations to your vehicle. Insurers will want to know about any disabilities or health problems, particularly if there have been any restrictions imposed on your licence. Insurers are not allowed to refuse insurance to disabled drivers unless they can justify it. Any insurance premium has to be based on a reasonable assessment of risk.

If you feel that an insurer has behaved unreasonably or has not acted within the remit of the Equality Act 2010 (see Parkinson's and employment) you should complain directly to the insurer. If the response of the Insurer is not satisfactory then you should go to the Financial Services Ombudsman (address at the back of the book).

Adaptations to vehicles for drivers with Parkinson's

If you have Parkinson's and it is impacting on your driving comfort and safety, then you can get your vehicle adapted to suit your particular condition. There are motoring accessories available for people with upper or lower body disabilities or both, which include:

- Hand controls to operate the accelerator or break
- Aids to help you turn the steering wheel with greater ease
- Accessories to help you get in and out of your vehicle such as cushions, covers and support
- Adapted mirrors for greater vision
- Different types of seat belts and harnesses
- Lifts and wheelchair hoists.

This list is not exclusive there are a number of adaptations which would be recommended at the time of fitting.

Dropped kerbs

A dropped kerb can make it easier to access your vehicle. For this you would normally apply to your local county council (or your local authority who can advise). More information is available on the DirectGov website.

****

Chapter 12

People who care for Parkinson's Sufferer's

Definition of a carer

We have all heard of the word "carer". This denotes a number of things. A carer can be someone who looks after their mother or father or looks after someone else in the family or a friend in an unpaid capacity. A carer is quite different to a home help.

Someone who is in the position of a carer for a person who has been diagnosed with Parkinson's can claim benefits in certain circumstances, access help and support from social services and also receive priority support from local health services. Carer's benefits are outlined in the chapter on welfare benefits.

Providing care to a person with Parkinson's

As the symptoms associated with Parkinson's will change over time, the nature of the care that is provided will also, of necessity, change with that person's needs. For example, in the early stages of Parkinson's the level of care needed may be minimal. It is at this early stage that it is important to gather as much information as you possibly can about the condition so you can become acquainted with the possible future needs of the person. You can gather information from a number of sources, the Internet, for example from Parkinson's UK www.parkinsons.org.uk or from medical and social services providers.

Many people with Parkinson's stay independent for years after their initial diagnosis and won't really need a lot of care. It is important during this time to display a positive attitude which can be of great benefit to your partner or relative/friend and can make a significant difference to how they cope with Parkinson's. There are a number of ways that you as a carer can assist, such as encouraging them to lead as active and normal a life as is possible under the circumstances and allowing them to do as much for themselves as possible.

If you feel that you need further training and advice in this area there are a number of courses, and informal groupings, available for carer's which explore the issues involved and allow you to meet other people in the same circumstances. There are useful contacts listed at the end of this chapter and at the back of the book.

Talking to health professionals

Your GP will be the first person you should talk to about your caring responsibilities. Carer's are given special consideration because of their role and the pressure that comes with that role. It always helps to compile a list of your needs and of the concerns that you wish to discuss with your doctor. Again, Parkinson's UK has useful information relating to discussing things with your doctor.

Following discussions with your GP, he/she will then, through the primary care team provide support and advice and:

- Arrange home visits to you or the person that you care for
- Arrange appointments for you and the person that you care for at the same time
- Supply repeat prescriptions to be delivered to your local pharmacy
- Put you in touch with other sources of support and advice such as other voluntary advice agencies
- Provide any letters of support that may be required for benefit departments or other agencies, such as the Blue Badge Scheme.

The Carer's Register

A carer's register is a database compiled by (some) surgeries that will enable staff to identify carer's and also those in receipt of care. The register is used to help get the right services at the right time, provide clear information about other relevant services and receive up-to-date information about events for carer's. In addition, the register will ensure that appointments are offered at appropriate times and that outpatient appointments and letters make clear that the person is a carer.

Time off from caring

Time of from caring is known as a 'Respite Break'. Time off from caring responsibilities is very important. Taking a break can help alleviate the anxieties and depression that accompany the role of carer. Respite breaks don't always mean that you have to go away somewhere, they can be given in a variety of ways, such as a social services care worker taking over for a while, or someone from a charity such as Crossroads Care (address at the back of the book) coming to the home regularly to care for the person with Parkinson's. In addition, the person that you care for can spend some time at a day centre or can spend short periods in a care home. All of this will depend on the circumstances at the time.

Carer's assessments

The local authority in your area has responsibility for arranging services that can help you take a break from caring. This will be achieved through a carer's assessment. Social services then use the assessment to decide what services to provide. You would normally initiate the assessment by visiting the social services department of the local council and asking for an assessment for the person that you care for and also for yourself as the carer.

The social services department will also carry out a financial assessment, which may mean that either you or the person being cared for will be responsible for all or some of the services provided. The decision to charge will be according to means.

Carers and employment rights

We discussed carers rights in chapter ten, dealing with rights whilst in employment. If you are in the position where you are caring for someone with Parkinson's and also working at the same time, you may find that the pressure on you as a person increases significantly. Carer's have statutory rights at work that can help reduce this pressure and also help to meet other needs. Employers also may be able to offer additional flexibility through their own policies and procedures.

Telling your employer about your role as a carer

There is no legal obligation to inform your employer about your role as carer. If you decide to tell your employer then make sure that you are fully aware of your statutory rights. You can find detailed information about your rights and employer's responsibilities from Carers UK www.carersuk.org and DirectGov.

Statutory rights for carer's

The main law protecting carer's in the workplace is the Work and Families Act 2006 and the Employment Rights Act 1996, which give working carer's rights to help them manage work and caring. This includes the right to request flexible work and leave entitlement. In Northern Ireland they are called the Work and Families (Northern Ireland) Order 2006 and the Employment Rights (Northern Ireland) Order 2006. Your employment status can affect your entitlement to statutory rights. If you are self-employed, on a short term contract or employed through an agency you may not be covered by these rights. If this applies to you, contact ACAS on 08457 47 47 47 for further advice.

Your employer may already have procedures in place to support carer's. This will usually be within the staff handbook or the intranet. The size and nature of the employer will determine whether or not they have publicized these rights. The public sector or large private sector employers are usually better at doing this.

As a working carer, you are likely to need a range of support, from access to a telephone to leave arrangements that work around the hospital visits etc of the person with Parkinson's.

You have a right to a ' reasonable' amount of time off work to deal with an emergency involving a dependant, such as a disruption or breakdown in care arrangements, a dependant falling ill or time to make better long term arrangements for a dependant. The right also includes some protection from victimisation or dismissal when you take time off. It is at the employer's discretion whether the leave is paid or unpaid.

Useful websites for carers to gain further information about the role of a carer and rights and responsibilities

Carers Direct www.nhs/carersdirect

Carers direct gives information and advice to carers

Care Directions www.caredirections.co.uk

Care Directions gives advice and information on health and care issues for older people

Carers Federation www.carersfederation.co.uk

The Carers Federation provides support for carers and for others with medical and mental health issues.

Carers UK www.carersuk.org

Carers UK is the main voice of carers in the UK providing advice and information and also campaigning on behalf of carers.

Crossroads care www.crossroads.org.uk

Crossroads provides support for carers and those being cared for.

Disabled Living Foundation www.dlf.org.uk

The Disabled Living foundation is a charity that provides advice about disability aids.

Employers for carers www.employersforcarers.org

Employers for carers provides practical advice for employers concerning the support of carers in their workforce.

Relate www.relate.org.uk

Relate provides relationship counselling and support services.

Relatives and residents association www.relres.org

The Relatives and Residents association provides advice and information on care homes and support for those with emotional concerns.

The Outsiders www.outsiders.org.uk

The Outsiders is a social and peer support network of disabled people, offering advice for people who have concerns about sexual or personal relationships.

The Princess Royal Trust for Carers www.carers.org

The Princess royal trust offers information and support for carers.

Young Carers Initiative www.youngcarer.com

The Young Carers Initiative offers advice and support to young carers and their families.

****

Useful Addresses

Ability Net Central England
PO Box 94
Warwick
Warwickshire.
CV34 5WS
Freephone: 0800 269545
Web: www.abilitynet.org.uk

Information on specialist assistive technology to help people with
Any disability to use a computer.

Advisory, Conciliation and Arbitration Service (ACAS)
Helpline 08457 47 47 47
www.acas.org.uk

Provides information to both employers and employees seeking
information on employment rights and obligations.

Access to Work (England, Scotland and Wales)
London (for South East England and East England)
atwosu.london.dwp.gsi.gov.uk
Tel: 020 8426 3133

Cardiff (for South West England, Wales, West Midlands and East
Midlands)
atwosu.london.dwp.gsi.gov.uk
Tel: 02920 423 291

Glasgow (for Scotland, North West England, North East England,
Yorkshire and Humberside)
atwosu.glasgow@dwp.gsi.gov.uk
Tel: 0141 950 5327

Age UK
Astral house
1268 London Road
London
SW16 4ER
Tel: 020 8765 7200
Helpline: 0800 009966
www.age.uk.org.uk

Researches into the needs of elderly
People and is involved in policy-making.

Benefits Enquiry Line
Tel: 0800 882200
Minicom: 0800 243355
www.dwp.gov.uk
N. Ireland 0800 220674

Warbreck House
Warbreck Hill Road
Blackpool
FY2 0YE
Email: bel-customer-services@dwp.gsi.gov.uk

Government agency giving information and
Advice on sickness and disability benefits for
People with disabilities and their carers.

British Association / College of
Occupational Therapists
106-114 Borough High Street
London
SE1 1LB

Tel:020 7357 6480 or
020 7450 2330
www.cot.org.uk

Information about all aspects of Occupational
Therapy. An S.A.E. requested.

Carers UK
20 Great Dover Street
London
SE1 4LX
Tel: 020 7378 4 999
Carers' line: 0808 808 7777
www.carersuk.org

Offers information and support to all people
Who are unpaid carers, looking after others
With medical or other problems.

Chartered Society of Physiotherapy
14 Bedford Row
London
WC1R 4ED
Tel:020 7306 6666
www.csp.org.uk
Information about all aspects of physiotherapy.

Citizens Advice Bureaux
(National Association of CABs)
Myddelton House
115-123 Pentonville Road
London
N1 9LZ

0844 411 1444
www.citizensadvice.org.uk

HQ of national charity offering a wide variety of practical and legal advice. Network of local branches throughout the UK listed in phone books and Yellow Pages under Counselling and Advice.

Counsel and Care
Twyman House
Bonny Street
London
NW1 9PG
Tel: 020 7241 8555
Helpline: 0845 300 7585
(Mon-Fri 10am-4pm except Wed 10am-1pm)
www.counselandcare.org.uk

Information and advice on homes,community
Care and housing with care.

Crossroads Caring for Carers
10 Regent Place
Rugby
Warwickshire
CV21 2PN
Helpline: 0845 450 0350
www.crossroads.org.uk

Supports and delivers high-quality service for
Carers and people with care needs via its local branches.

Dial UK
St Catherine's

Tickhill Road
Doncaster
S. Yorkshire
DN4 8QN
Tel / texphone: 01302 310123
www.dialuk.info

Nationwide network offering information and
Advice on all aspects of disability ; 130 drop -in
Centres run by and for people with disabilities.

Disability Law Service
Tel: 020 7791 9800
www.dls.org.uk

This organisation provides specialist legal advice for disabled people,
their families and carers.

Disability Action (Northern Ireland)
Tel: 028 9029 7880
www.disabilityaction.org

This organisation works to ensure that people with disabilities attain
their full rights as citizens, by supporting inclusion, influencing
government policy and changing attitudes in partnership with
disabled people.

Disabled Living Foundation
380-384 Harrow Road
London
W9 2HU
Tel: 020 7289 6111
Helpline: 0845 130 9177

www.dlf.org.uk

Provides information to disabled and elderly people
On all kinds of equipment in order to promote
Their independence and quality of life.

DVLA
Driver and Vehicle Licensing Agency
Swansea
SA6 7JL
Tel: 0870 600 0301
www.dvla.gov.uk

Provides information about
Medical conditions, driving licences, learning
To drive, entitlement to drive

Equality Advisory Support Service (EASS)
Tel: 0808 800 0084
www.equalityadvisoryservice.com

Equality and Human Rights Commission
www.equalityhumanrights.com

European Parkinson's Disease Association
(EPDA)
1 Northumberlad Avenue
Trafalgar Square
London WC2N 5BW
Tel: 0207 872 5510
www.epda.eu.com

Umbrella body for network of international
Parkinson's disease groups, campaigning on behalf
Of all suffers. Information leaflets on request.
An S.A.E. requested.

Homecraft Rolyan
Nunn Brook Road
Huthwaite
Sutton in Ashfield
Notts
NG17 2HU
Tel: 0844 412 4330
(For International Visitors
Tel: +44 1623 448706)
www.homecraft-rolyan.com

Mail order company offering a wide range of items and equipment
suitable for people with disabilities.

Institute for Complementary and
Natural Medicine
Can- Mezzanine
32-36 Loman Street
London
SE1 0EH
Tel: 08454 456 2537
www.i-c-m.org.uk

Umbrella group for complementary medicine organisation. Offers
information, safe choice to Public.

Keep Able
3-4 Sterling Park

Pedmore Road
Brierley Hill
W. Midlands
DY51 1TB
Tel: 0870 520 2122 or
Tel: 084 4888 1338
Fax: 013 8448 0260
www.keepable.co.uk

Nationwide chain of stores, advising
And suppling a wide range of products
For people with disabilities.

Leonard Cheshire Disability
66 South Lambeth Road
London
SW8 1RL
Tel: 020 3242 0200
www.lcdisability.org
Email: info@lcdisability.org
Contact Customer Helpline on 0808 808 2236
email customerhelpline@lcdisability.org

Nation offices
Leonard Cheshire Disability Scotland
Murrayburgh House
17 Corstorphine Road
Edinburgh
EH12 6DD
Tel: 0131 346 9040
Fax: 0131 346 9050
email: scotlandoffice@LCDisability.org

Leonard Cheshire Disability Wales
Centre for Business
Office 3
12 Devon Place
Newport
Gwent
NP20 4NN
Tel: 01633 263807

Leonard Cheshire Disability Northern Ireland
5 Boucher Plaza
4-6 Boucher Road
Belfast
BT12 6HR
Tel: 028 9024 6247
Fax: 028 9024 6395
email: northernirelandoffice@LCDisability.org

Offers care, support and a wide range of Information for disabled people aged between 18 and 65 years in the UK and worldwide to encourage independent living. Has respite and residential homes; offers holidays and rehabilitation.

Mobilise
National HQ
Ashwellthorpe
Norwich
NR16 1EX
Tel: 01508 489449
www.mobilise.info

Provides information for drivers with a disability on a wide range of issues.

Motability
Motability Operations
City Gate House
22 Southwark Bridge Road
London
SE1 9HB
Tel:0845 456 4566
www.motability.co.uk

Helps driver with disabilities to access specialist
Cars and funding with Motability car schemes.

**National Institute for Health and Clinical
Excellence (NICE)**
MidCity Place
71 High Holborn
London
WC1V 6NA
Tel: 0845 003 7780
www.nice.org.uk

Provides national guidance on the
Promotion of good health and treatment
of ill-health. Patient information leaflets
Are available for each piece of guidance issued.

NHS Direct
Tel: 0845 4647 (24 hours, 365days a year)
www.nhsdirect.nhs.uk

Parkinson's UK
National Office

215 Vauxhall Bridge Road
London
Hepline: 0808 800 0303
Tel: 020 7931 8080
Fax: 020 7233 9908
www.parkinsons.org.uk
Email: hello@parkinsons.org.uk

Northern Ireland office
Parkinson's UK Northern Ireland
Wellington Park Business Centre
3 Wellington Park
Malone Road
Belfast BT9 6DJ
Phone: 028 9092 3370
Email: northernireland@parkinsons.org.uk

Scotland office
Parkinson's UK Scotland
Forsyth House
Lomond Court
Castle Business Park
Stirling FK9 4TU
Phone: 01786 433811
Email: scotland@parkinsons.org.uk

Wales office
Parkinson's UK Wales/Cymru
Maritime Offices
Woodland Terrace
Maesycoed
Pontypridd CF37 1DZ
Phone: 0844 225 3784

Email: wales@parkinsons.org.uk
Offers information and support via its local groups Has nurse specialists and welfare department, And funds research into Parkinson's disease.

Patients' Association
PO Box 935
Harrow
Middlesex
HA1 3YJ
Helpline: 0845 608 4455
Tel: 020 8423 9111
www.patients-association.com
Email: helpline@patients-association.com

Provides advice on patients' rights, leaflets and
A directory of self-help groups.

Disability Rights UK
12 City Forum
250 City Road
London
EC1V 8AF
Tel: 020 7250 3222
www. disabilityrightsuk

Campaigns to improve the rights and care of disabled people. Sells special key to access locked disabled toilets.

Royal College of Speech and Language
Therapy
2 White Hart Yard
London

SE1 1NX
Tel: 020 7378 1200
www.rcslt.org

Information about all aspects of speech
And language therapy.

Vitalise
212 Business Design centre
52 Upper street
London N1 OQH
General Enquiries 0303 303 0145

Provides information to people with disabilities on transport,
holiday accommodation, activity holidays are respite care
establishments in the UK and abroad .

YPN (Younger Parkinson's Network)
National helpline : 0808 800 0303

The young-onset self-help group of Parkinson's UK and is designed
really for those of working age. There are around 1,300 members of
YPN , many of them in their early 20s and 30s. Has a magazine,
local meetings and conference every 2 years.

Parkinson's UK Support Group
Townsend Hall
Shipston on Stour
Warks
CV36 4AE
Tel: 0844 225 3644
www.parkinson.org.uk

David Rayner Centre
120 Cambridge Road
Great Shelford
Cambridege
CB22 5JT
Helpline: 080 8800 0303
www.parkinsons.org.uk

Network of local groups bringing people with Parkinson's and their families together for support and help.

Parkinson's Home Care
Helping Hand Homecare
Arrow House
8-9 Church Street
Alcester
Warwickshire
B49 5AJ
Free phone: 0808 180 9455
www.helpinghandscare.co.uk

Specific Information for drivers

Driving and Parkinson's
Association of British Insurers (ABI) www.abi.org.uk

The ABI will assist you with any complaints that you may have about insurers

Department for Transport www.dft.gov.uk

The DFT aims to ensure that provisions for all motorists are acceptable, accessible and affordable.

Disability Alliance www.disability alliance.org

The Disability Alliance provides advice on benefits and services for people with disabilities.

Disabled Living Foundation www.dlf.org.uk

As above provides advice and information.

DVLA (Driver and Vehicle Licensing Agency) www.dvla.gov.uk

The DVLA will provide advice and information on all aspects of driving.

Mobilise www.mobilise.info

Mobilise provides help and support to disabled drivers and passengers.

Motability www.motability.co.uk
Motability helps to keep disabled drivers on the road.

Appendix 1
Sample medication log

As mentioned earlier in the chapter on finding and dealing with doctors and specialists, it is very important to keep a log of the medications that you take and when you take them, plus also the types of symptoms that you are experiencing. The below is an example which might help you.

Medication

Date	Time	Type and dosage	Symptoms/moods	Next dose

24 Hour record of symptoms

Date_____

Time	Medication dosage	Symptoms/moods
6am		
8am		
10am		
12noon		
2pm		
4pm		
6pm		
8pm		
10pm		
12am		
2am		
4am		

The purpose of the logs on the previous page is to ensure that you have an accurate record of what exactly is happening to you in order that both your doctor and anyone who interacts with you on a professional level understands and knows what is going on. As stated, it is likely that your doctor will have an accurate record, as this is their job, but others who deal with you may not.

****

Index

Emerald Publishing
www.emeraldpublishing.co.uk

Other titles in the Emerald Series:

Law
Guide to Bankruptcy
Conducting Your Own Court case
Guide to Consumer law
Creating a Will
Guide to Family Law
Guide to Employment Law
Guide to European Union Law
Guide to Health and Safety Law
Guide to Criminal Law
Guide to Landlord and Tenant Law
Guide to the English Legal System
Guide to Housing Law
Guide to Marriage and Divorce
Guide to The Civil Partnerships Act
Guide to The Law of Contract
The Path to Justice
You and Your Legal Rights
The Debt Collecting Merry Go Round
Powers of Attorney

Health
Guide to Combating Child Obesity
Asthma Begins at Home
Explaining Bipolar Disorder

The Ultimate Nutrition Guide for Cancer Sufferers and Their Friends and Family
The Ultimate Nutrition Guide for Osteoporosis Sufferers
The Sea Medicine Chest
Natures Aspirin

Music
How to Survive and Succeed in the Music Industry

General
A Practical Guide to Obtaining probate
A Practical Guide to Residential Conveyancing
Writing The Perfect CV
Keeping Books and Accounts-A Small Business Guide
Business Start Up-A Guide for New Business
Finding Asperger Syndrome in the Family-A Book of Answers
Writing Your Autobiography
Being a professional Writer

For details of the above titles published by Emerald go to:

www.emeraldpublishing.co.uk